Pocket Guide to
Physical Assessment

Pocket Guide to
Physical Assessment

Patricia A. Potter, RN, MSN

Director of Nursing Practice
Barnes Hospital
St. Louis, Missouri

SECOND EDITION

with 61 *illustrations*

The C. V. Mosby Company

St. Louis · Baltimore · Philadelphia · Toronto   1990

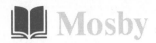

Editor Nancy L. Coon
Developmental Editors Susan R. Epstein, Suzanne Seeley
Project Manager Patricia Tannian
Production Editor Tim Sainz
Design Rey Umali

Printed in the United States of America

The C.V. Mosby Company
11830 Westline Industrial Drive, St. Louis, Missouri 63146

Library of Congress Cataloging in Publication Data
Potter, Patricia Ann.
  Pocket guide to physical assessment / Patricia A. Potter.—2nd ed.
    p. cm.
  Rev. ed. of: Pocket nurse guide to physical assessment. 1986.
  Includes bibliographical references.
  ISBN 0-8016-3377-X
  1. Nursing assessment—Handbooks, manuals, etc. 2. Physical
diagnosis—Handbooks, manuals, etc. I. Potter, Patricia Ann.
Pocket nurse guide to physical assessment.
  [DNLM: 1. Nursing Process—handbooks. 2. Physical Examination—
handbooks. 3. Physical Examination—nurse's instruction. WY 39
P868p)
RT48.P68   1990
616.07′54—dc20
DNLM/DLC   90-5469
for Library of Congress   CIP

C/D/D   9   8   7   6   5   4   3   2

Preface

The nursing assessment is the process of gathering, verifying, analyzing, and communicating data about a client. The purpose of the assessment is to establish a database about the client's level of wellness, health practices, past illnesses and related experiences, and health care goals. The database is derived from a nursing health history, physical examination, and the results of laboratory and diagnostic test results. The information contained in the database is the basis for an individualized plan of nursing care that is developed throughout the nursing process.

The *Pocket Guide to Physical Assessment,* second edition, is a useful guide for nurses performing physical assessments in any type of clinical setting. The organization of the guide provides a quick reference when the practicing nurse's assessment focuses on a specific body system. However, the guide can also be used when the nurse wishes to conduct a complete physical examination.

Features of the guide include a summary of client and equipment preparation, a step-by-step approach to body system assessment, a review of normal and abnormal findings of the adult, special gerontologic and pediatric factors the nurse should consider during assessment, and a "nurse alert" section that cautions the nurse about techniques to avoid or symptoms to be alert for during an examination.

Patricia A. Potter

Contents

Part II   **Measurement of Vital Signs**

6   **Body Temperature,** 45

PART I

PRELIMINARY
SKILLS

Physical Assessment in Nursing Practice

Nursing, as defined in the American Nurses' Association (ANA) social policy statement, is "the diagnosis and treatment of human responses to actual or potential health problems" (ANA, 1980). A nurse uses clinical skills and theoretical knowledge to interpret clinical situations and make decisions about a client's care. Information gathered through a nursing history and physical assessment allows a nurse to make clinical judgments through the formulation of nursing diagnoses of collaborative health problems. Focusing on a client's diagnoses and health problems gives the nurse clear direction in selecting client goals and nursing interventions.

Nursing Diagnosis

A nursing diagnosis is a clinical judgment made by a professional nurse about an individual, family, or community. It is derived through a deliberate systematic process of data collection and analysis (Shoemaker, 1984). A nursing diagnosis has three essential components, known as PES (Gordon, 1976):

P—Health problems or status of an individual, family, or community. Diagnoses such as pain, knowledge deficit, and body image disturbance are short, clear, precise statements. Actual or potential problems may be diagnosed.

E—Related or etiologic factors contribute to the existence or maintenance of a client's health problems. Related factors are assessed as either internal or external to the client. Selection of a related or causal factor helps nurses focus on nursing interventions that are most appropriate to meet a client's goals of care. At times there may be more than one related factor for a diagnosis. Singling out one related

Table 1   Sample nursing diagnoses

Defining Characteristics	Nursing Diagnosis	Related Factors
Verbalizes history of pain for less than 6 months	Acute pain	Traumatic injury
Vocalizes presence of sharp, tingling pain in right shoulder		
Restlessness		
Facial grimacing during shoulder movement		
Newly diagnosed as having diabetes	Knowledge deficit	Newly diagnosed disease
Unable to explain or discuss nature of disease		Unfamiliarity with disease process
Questions the significance of diabetes and its implications		
Wife shows interest in the client's problems		

factor may inhibit a nurse's holistic approach to care. Use of a nursing diagnosis alone can be sufficient and provide direction for planning care without narrowing the focus to only one aspect of a more complex health problem (McFarland, 1989).

S—The final component in the structural definition of nursing diagnosis is the defining characteristics. These are the subjective and objective signs and symptoms indicating the presence of a condition that corresponds to a given nursing diagnosis (Table 1). The nurse must use clinical reasoning to cluster the data collected and formulate the most appropriate diagnosis.

Collaborative Problems

Nurses do not care for clients by themselves. A significant part of a nurse's practice is in collaboration with other health care professionals such as physicians. For example, a client may have a medical diagnosis of coronary artery disease. Collaborative problems that require the nurse's ongoing assessment include potential risks for cardiac dysrhythmias or anginal attacks. However, pertinent nursing diagnoses for this same client might include "knowledge deficit regarding disease process" or "activity intolerance related to oxygen imbalance."

Collaborative problems require a nurse to monitor a client's condition. However, any orders specific to treating the problems are initiated by a physician. The nurse carries out orders for treatment but consults with the physician when changes occur and new orders become necessary. Collaborative problems are just as important as nursing diagnoses, but they represent the interdependent role of nursing, whereas nursing diagnoses represent nursing's independent role (Carpenito, 1986). Nursing diagnoses are holistic and thus may be used to describe problems of a physiologic, psychologic, developmental, social, or spiritual problem. In contrast, medical diagnoses are made principally of physiologic or psychologic alterations. The skills of physical assessment are used regardless of the type of problem a nurse must assess or evaluate.

Nursing History: Tips and Techniques

2

The nursing history obtained during an interview with a client is normally conducted before the physical assessment. The history is the data collected about a client's level of wellness, changes in life patterns, sociocultural roles, and mental and emotional reactions to illness. Incorporating data from the major health dimensions into a nursing history allows the nurse to develop a complete plan of care. When taking a health history, the nurse uses interviewing skills to gather a complete and accurate database that helps the nurse focus attention during the physical assessment on select body systems or symptoms.

Models for Data Collection

Nurses use a variety of approaches when collecting a nursing health history. In acute care settings the model or format used may be that found in the institution's admission or history form (Fig. 1). It is important, however, for the nurse to use a model that captures all data relevant to a client's health status. Most models contain basic components similar to the following model:

- Biographic information, which should include date of birth, sex, the names of close family members or significant others, marital status, religious preference, occupation, and source of health care insurance
- Reasons for seeking health care, which should include goals of care and expectations of services and treatment
- Present illness or health concern, which should include information about the onset of concern, symptoms, nature and duration of symptoms, precipitating factors, and relief measures

BARNES

NURSE ADMISSION NOTE

Date _____ Time _____ Informant _____ *Age _____

T ____ P ____ R ____ B/P _____ Ht. ____ Wt. ____

Chief Complaint and History of Present Illness:

ADDRESSOGRAPH

Medical/Surgical History	Date

Medical/Surgical History	Date

Has received blood products in the past: ☐ Yes ☐ No   If yes, list dates _____

Reactions: ☐ Yes ☐ No

Allergies: _____

Medication Name	Dose/Frequency	Time of Last Dose

Medication Name	Dose/Frequency	Time of Last Dose

Continued.

Fig. 1
Dimensions for gathering data for health history.

Patient Provided: ☐ Admission Kit ☐ ID Band ☐ Sensitivity/Allergy Band ☐ Sensitivity/Allergy Sticker on Chart
Patient Instructed: ☐ Valuables Policy ☐ Waiver Signed ☐ Smoking/Visitor Policy ☐ Nurses Call/Emergency/TV/Phone
☐ Chaplain Availability ☐ Patient Rights (Psych. Only)

SIGNATURE: _____

Directions: Assess each standard on admission. If unable to assess within 24 hours, explain. S = Subjective   O = Objective

Sensory
- S: *Vision/ *Hearing problems   Glasses   Contacts   Prosthesis   Hearing aid
- O: Discharge: Eyes/Ears/Nose   Numbness   Tingling   Decreased sensation

Sensory Alterations

Comments:

Skin/Mucous Membrane
- S: Lesions   Itching   Change in skin color
- O: Break in skin integrity   Wound   Pressure ulcer   Lesions   Body secretions/excretions
  Condition of mouth _____

Impaired Skin Integrity
Alt in Oral Mucous Membrane

Comments:

Respiratory
- S: Cough   SOB   Sputum production   Uses home O2 _____ L/min.
- O: Lung sounds   Confusion   Restlessness

Ineffective Airway Clearance
Ineffective Breathing Pattern
Impaired Gas Exchange

Comments:

Circulatory
- S: *Fatigue   *Lightheadedness   Slow healing of lesion   Leg cramps   Edema   Chest pain
- O: Extremities (color/temperature/pulses)

Decreased Cardiac Output
Alt. Periph. Tissue Perfusion
Alt. Fluid Volume

Comments:

Nutrition
- S: Decreased/Increased appetite   Difficulty chewing   Dysphagia   N or V
  Dentures: (lower/upper/partial)   Current diet: _____   Recent weight gain/loss: _____

Alt. in Nutrition

- O:

Comments:

Elimination

Alt. in Bowel Elimination
Alt. in Urinary Elimination

- S: Hemorrhoids   *Diarrhea   Constipation   Abd. pain   Cramps   Gas
  Usual pattern _____   Last BM _____   Use of enemas/Laxatives _____
  *Frequency   *Urgency   Incontinence   Polyuria   Dysuria   Hematuria   *Nocturia   Retention
  Bowel sounds _____   Urine _____   Ostomy (Bowel/Urinary) _____
- O: _____
- Comments:

Activity/Exercise

Impaired Physical Mobility
Self-care Deficit
Activity Intolerance

- S: *Fatigue   Exertional discomfort or SOB   *Decreased strength   *Fall Hx   *Abnormal gait
  *Impaired coordination   Assistive devices _____
- O: *ROM _____   *Weight bearing _____
  *Self-care limitations/ *disabilities _____
- Comments:

Comfort

Alt. in Comfort
Alt. in Sleep Pattern

- S: Pain: _____   Comfort Measures: _____
  *Sleep disturbances _____   Sleeping aids _____
- O: Behaviors indicating pain or sleep problems _____
- Comments:

Immune Function

Potential for infection

- S: Chronic disease   Transplant   Radiation   Chemotherapy   Steroids
- O: Broken skin   Invasive device
- Comments:

Sexuality/Reproductive

Alt. in Sexual Function/
Response

- S: LMP _____   Pregnant _____   Family Planning Method _____
  Breast massess/tenderness   Prostate enlargment   Vaginal/Urethral/Breast discharge   STD
  Concern about sexual functioning R/T disease/therapy   Concern about relationship with partner
- Comments:

Fig. 1, cont'd.
For legend see p. 7.

Continued.

Neuro Cerebral Function

Alt. in Thought Processes
Alt. in Communication
Potential for Violence

- S: Family report of change in behavior _____ *Impaired memory / *Attention span / *Judgment / *Perception
- O: Alert   *Oriented x _____
- Comments: _____

Cognitive Response

Lack of Knowledge

- S: Inexperience with therapy/disease/hospitalization
- O: Asks questions   Requests information   Barriers to learning (*langauge/vision/hearing/literacy) _____
  Identified needs for teaching/teaching aids: _____
- Comments: _____

Emotional Response

Alt. in Coping
Alt. in Self-Concept
Fear
Anxiety
Dysfunctional Grieving

- S: Low mood   Fear   Chronic worry   Loss of control   Inability to cope or problem solve
- O: *Alcohol / *Drug Abuse   Smoker (packs per day _____)
  Anxious   Angry   Apprehensive   Crying   Irritable   Self-neglect   Lack of eye contact
  Loss or change in structure/function of body part
- Comments: _____

Social System

Alt. in Family Processes
Social Isolation

- S: Occupation _____   Retired (former work) _____
  Lives: Home   ECF   Alone   With family   Support person: _____
  Feeling of aloneness/rejection/being different from others
  Family unable to meet physical/emotional/spiritual needs   Home environment affecting care: _____
- Comments: _____

Value/Beliefs

Spiritual Distress

- S: Attitudes/beliefs re: hospitalization/implications of care _____
  Perceptions of illness (patient/family) _____
  Questions suffering/concern with meaning of life/death/belief system _____
- Comments: _____

Health Management

Pattern

Alt. in Health Maintenance

Potential for Injury

• S: Last physical _____   Last pap smear _____   Mammogram _____

Performs self-breast exam/testicular exam _____   Exercise Program _____

*Non-compliance with restrictions/therapies _____   Use of *tranquilizers/ *narcotics/ *multiple medications

Needs equipment/finances/resources _____

• O: *Risk factors for injury _____

Comments: _____

_____

_____

RN Signature: _____   Date: _____   Time: _____

Reviewed by: _____   Date: _____   Time: _____

140996 REV. 6/89

*Factors for fall risk evaluation

Fig. 1, cont'd.
For legend see p. 7.

- Past health history, which should include previous illnesses throughout client's development, injuries and hospitalizations, surgeries, blood transfusions, allergies, immunizations, habits such as use of cigarettes, caffeine, alcohol and other drugs, prescribed or self-prescribed medications, and patterns of sleep, exercise, and eating
- Family history, which should include health status of the immediate family and living blood relations, cause of death of blood relatives, and risk-factor analysis for cancer, heart disease, diabetes mellitus, hypertension, and mental disorders
- Environmental history, which should include information about exposure to hazards and pollutants and physical safety
- Psychosocial and cultural history, which should include primary language, cultural group, community resources, mood, attention span, and developmental stage
- Review of systems, which should include a head-to-toe review of all major body systems, as well as client's knowledge of and compliance with health care (for example, last visual acuity exam)

Functional Health Patterns

One model that has gained acceptance in health assessment is Marjory Gordon's functional health pattern framework (1987). The model is organized by functional health patterns that make it useful in collecting data to formulate nursing diagnoses. The framework can be used for clients of all ages and in assessment of families and communities. Gordon's model is summarized in the following list:

- Health-Perception–Health-Management Pattern describes clients' perceived pattern of health and well-being and how their health is managed
- Nutritional-Metabolic Pattern describes consumption relative to metabolic need and nutrient supply; includes pattern of food and fluid consumption, condition of skin, hair, nails, and mucous membranes, body temperature, height, and weight
- Elimination Pattern describes patterns of excretory function (bowel, bladder, and skin); includes individual's daily pattern, changes or disturbances, and methods used to control excretion
- Activity-Exercise Pattern describes pattern of exercise, activ-

ity, leisure, and recreation; includes activities of daily living, type and quality of exercise, and factors affecting pattern (such as neuromuscular, respiratory, and circulatory)

- Sleep-Rest Pattern describes pattern of sleep, rest, and relaxation and any aids to change those patterns
- Cognitive-Perceptual Pattern describes sensory-perceptual and cognitive pattern; includes adequacy of sensory modes (vision, hearing, touch, taste, and smell), reports of pain perception, and cognitive functional abilities
- Self-Perception–Self-Concept Pattern describes self-concept pattern and perceptions of self
- Role Relationship Pattern describes pattern of role engagements and relationships; includes perception of major roles and responsibilities in current life situation
- Sexuality-Reproductive Pattern describes patterns of satisfaction or dissatisfaction with sexuality; includes female's reproductive state
- Coping–Stress Tolerance Pattern describes general coping pattern and effectiveness of the pattern in terms of stress tolerance
- Value-Belief Pattern describes patterns of values, goals, or beliefs (including spiritual beliefs) that guide choices or decisions

Guidelines for Collecting a Nursing History

- Assessment data sources should include the client, family or significant other, health team members, and the client's health record.
- Much data in the nursing history are subjective; the nurse should not challenge this information but should explore it with the client to clarify any vagueness and should record it as subjective data rather than objective data.
- When the client is critically ill, disoriented, confused, mentally handicapped, or very young, the family or significant others are necessary sources of information for the nursing history.
- The nursing history focuses on data from all the client's dimensions so that the nurse can develop a holistic nursing care plan.
- The recording of data in the nursing history should be clear and concise, using appropriate terminology.

Phases of the Interview

- Preparation. The nurse prepares by reviewing available information about the client in the medical record. At times this may be limited if the nurse is one of the first persons to see the client. The nurse also reviews literature related to the client's health problem. The interview should take place in a comfortable, quiet setting when possible.
- Orientation phase. The nurse explains the purpose of the interview and becomes acquainted with the client. Clarification is given regarding confidentiality of information. The nurse's professional approach evokes the client's trust. The nurse helps the client resolve any anxiety, feelings of helplessness, and concerns about the personal nature of information to be shared.
- Working phase. The nurse focuses the interview on the client's health dimensions, using a model that forms a database for eventual nursing diagnosis identification. The nurse uses interviewing skills to clarify and validate information so that appropriate clinical problem solving takes place. Data collected are later confirmed by findings from the physical examination. The nurse and client work together to identify problems and select goals of care.
- Termination phase. The nurse closes the interview by summarizing information collected. Problems or diagnoses and goals of care are validated with the client. The nurse explains how additional contact will be made with the client, including preparation for the physical assessment.

Interview Techniques

While collecting a nursing history, the nurse uses certain interviewing techniques that depend on the client's personality and health care needs.

- The problem-seeking technique uses questions to identify health problems the client needs to resolve.
- The problem-solving technique focuses on gathering more in-

formation about specific identified problems, such as onset of symptoms, aggravating factors, and attempted relief measures.

■ The direct-question technique is a more structured approach in which the client gives brief answers to factual types of questions.

■ The open-ended question technique fully explores the client's subjective symptoms and feelings with the client taking an active role in responding to questions that are phrased for full discussion.

Regardless of the interview technique used there are also the following basic communication strategies that the nurse uses to gather accurate and complete information:

Silence—allows the client to organize thoughts and present complete information

Attentive listening—shows the nurse's interest and concern and helps ensure that accurate data are collected

Conveying acceptance—communicates a willingness to listen nonjudgmentally

Related questions—focuses the interview on particular health issues or body systems to prevent rambling

Paraphrasing—provides an opportunity for the nurse to validate in more specific terms what the client has said

Clarifying—asking the client to restate information in more specific or other terms helps ensure that data are communicated correctly

Focusing—helps eliminate vagueness in communication by directing follow-up questions to the client to complete data

Stating observations—allows the client to receive feedback and encourages the client to offer additional pertinent information

Offering information—provides the client with health education, as appropriate

Summarizing—validates data from the client and signals the end of one part of the interview before continuing with the next part of the interview

Do's and Don'ts in Interviewing*

1. DO be assured of a quiet, private setting without distractions and interruptions.
2. DO use the most reliable source of information—if not the client, the closest family member.
3. DO use prior knowledge of diagnoses (if known) to plan information you want to focus on in obtaining the facts you need.
4. DO explain before starting that you will be asking many questions because you can provide better nursing care if you know more about the client and family.
5. DO write brief notations during your interview. Record dates, times, durations of hospitalizations, onsets of illness, and other data accurately. DON'T rely on memory. DON'T try to write finished sentences.
6. DO be calm, unhurried, and sympathetic. Show genuine interest and concern. (Sensitivity encourages the client to express feelings.) DON'T show annoyance or exasperation when the client hits a memory block. If you react with understanding, the client may recall the information later in a related question.
7. DO use eye contact appropriately. Observe facial expressions and body language. DON'T stare at the client or your outline.
8. DO use neutral, open-ended questions to elicit the verbalization of feelings and additional information. Use leading questions sparingly and judiciously— only for clarification of hazy comments. DO use the client's pertinent words to add to clarification. "By 'knifelike' pain, you mean sudden and intense?"
9. DO use terminology the client understands. If not sure whether the clients understand, ask what it means to them; or ask them to describe what the word means to them, for example, "Explain the 'nauseated feeling' you have."
10. DO ask about the client's complaints first to empha-

*From Eggland ET: How to take a meaningful nursing history, Nursing 77 7:22, 1977.

Do's and Don'ts in Interviewing—cont'd

size the purpose and expediency in your interviewing. DON'T start with delicate, personal questions.

11. DO allow the client to finish speaking, even if the statement is rambling. Then use direct questioning. DON'T continually jump between unrelated topics. DON'T repeat questions unnecessarily. If a repeat question is necessary, reword the question for better comprehension.

12. DO accept what the client says. A simple nod, um-hm, or glance will encourage the client to go on.

13. DO call the client by name. Express friendliness, pleasure, and concern. DON'T lose professional perspective or demeanor.

14. DO speak clearly, slowly, and distinctly.

15. DO listen.

Developmental Considerations

The nurse's approach to collecting a nursing history should consider the client's age.

Infants and Children

1. When obtaining histories for infants and children, gather all or part of the information from the parent or guardian.

2. Parents often think they are being tested by the interviewer. Offer support and do not pass judgment.

3. Use first names with children and honorific and last names with parents (for example, Mr. Smith).

4. If a young child becomes restless or uncooperative, divide the assessment into two sessions. Use of a toy, as well as the presence of parents, may have a calming effect.

5. Interviewing older children allows the nurse to observe parent-child interactions.

6. Adolescents tend to respond best when treated as adults and individuals.

7. Parents' reliability with information can vary. Concrete facts such as birth weight and birth date tend to be recalled most

accurately, minor illnesses tend to be forgotten more easily than are major ones, mothers of several children tend to be less accurate in their recall of most items than mothers of single children, and the mother's educational level is directly related to the accuracy of recall for some items, such as immunizations.

Elderly Adults

1. Do not stereotype aging clients. Most can adapt to change and learn about their health.
2. Sensory or physical limitations can affect how quickly the nurse can interview and later assess a client. Plan for more than one examination period.
3. Clients may find that giving certain types of health information is stressful; they may not discuss change or problems confirming their fear of illness or old age.
4. Data obtained depend on what the elderly client feels is important at the time.

Physical Assessment Skills

3

Four basic skills are used during the physical assessment: inspection, palpation, percussion, and auscultation. The specific uses of these skills are outlined in the assessment sections for the different body systems. The following sections summarize general principles for the use of these basic skills.

Inspection

Inspection is the use of vision, hearing, and smell to detect normal characteristics or significant physical signs of body parts.

- Inspection is the simplest technique to perform but is underused in physical assessment.
- Learn to recognize normal variations among clients, as well as ranges of normal in an individual.
- The examiner should be thorough and systematic in inspecting every body part.
- Good lighting and exposure are essential for careful inspection.
- Each body area is inspected for size, shape, color, position, symmetry with the opposite side of the body, and the presence of any abnormalities.
- Use additional light to inspect body cavities.
- Inspection is generally considered a visual skill but should include olfaction as well, since the sense of smell can sometimes detect abnormalities that may not be recognized by other means.

   Experience is generally the best guide in making judgments about odors detected during assessment.

   Ask a colleague to confirm your assessment if you are unsure about an odor.

Table 2   Assessment of characteristic odors

Odor	Site/Source	Potential Causes
Alcohol	Oral cavity	Ingestion of alcohol
Ammonia	Urine	Urinary tract infection
Body odor	Skin, particularly in areas where body parts rub together (under arms, beneath female breasts)	Poor hygiene, excess perspiration (hyperhidrosis), foul-smelling perspiration (bromidrosis)
Fecal odor	Wound site	Wound abscess
	Vomitus	Bowel obstruction
	Rectal area	Fecal incontinence
Foul-smelling stools (infant)	Stool	Malabsorption syndrome
Halitosis	Oral cavity	Poor dental and oral hygiene; gum disease
Sweet, fruity odor, ketones	Oral cavity	Diabetic acidosis
Stale urine odor	Skin	Uremic acidosis
Sweet, heavy, thick odor	Draining wound	*Pseudomonas* (bacterial) infection
Musty odor	Casted body part	Infection inside cast
Fetid, sweet odor	Tracheostomy or mucous secretions	Infection of bronchial tree (*Pseudomonas* bacteria)

Findings from olfaction should lead to more careful assessment of the body part or system with other assessment skills.

Table 2 lists common characteristic odors at different sites and their potential causes.

Palpation

Palpation is using the hands to touch body parts and make sensitive measurements of specific physical signs.

- Palpation is used to examine all accessible parts of the body, using different parts of the hand to detect characteristics of texture, shape, temperature, and movements (Fig. 2).
- Be sure client is relaxed and positioned comfortably to avoid muscle tension that may distort palpation findings.
- Palpate any known area of tenderness last.
- Keep fingernails short, warm hands before touching client, and use a gentle approach.

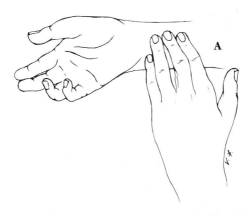

Fig. 2
A, Fingertips are the most sensitive parts of hand and are used to assess texture, shape, size, and consistency and for palpation. *Continued.*

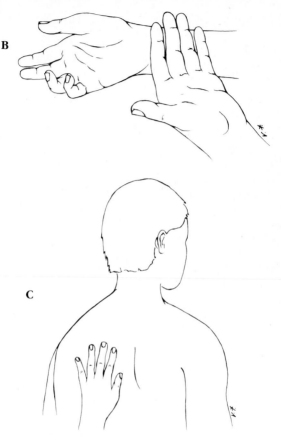

Fig. 2, cont'd.
B, Dorsum manus, or back of hand, is used to assess temperature. **C,** Palm of hand is sensitive to vibration.

- Apply tactile pressure in a slow, gentle, deliberate manner.
- Any tender areas should be examined further.
- The three methods of palpation are listed as follows (Fig. 3):
    Light palpation—fingers are gently applied over the skin surface; skin is depressed ½ to 1 cm (¼ to ½ inch).

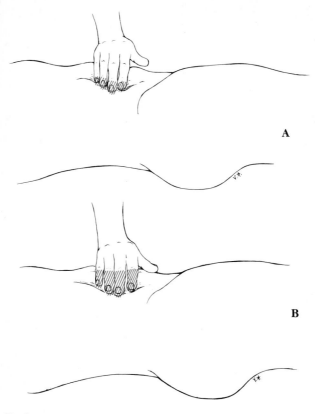

Fig. 3
The three techniques of palpation. **A,** Light palpation. **B,**
Deep palpation.   *Continued.*

Deep palpation—used to examine the condition of organs
and masses; skin is depressed 2 to 3 cm (1 to 1½ inches).
Caution is needed to prevent internal injury.
Bimanual palpation—both hands are used to palpate deeply;
one hand (the sensing hand) is relaxed and placed lightly on
the client's skin. The active hand applies pressure to the
sensing hand. The lower sensing hand remains sensitive to
detect organ characteristics.

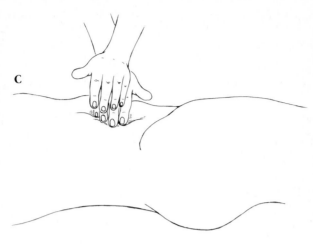

Fig. 3, cont'd.
C, Bimanual palpation.

- Palpation technique depends on the body area being examined and the client's condition, for example:

    With risk of a fractured rib, palpate with extreme care.

    When palpating a vital artery, avoid applying pressure that may obstruct the blood flow.

- Characteristics measured by palpation in major body areas are as follows:

Area of Body Examined	Criteria Measured by Palpation
Skin	Temperature
	Moisture
	Texture
	Turgor and elasticity
	Tenderness
	Thickness
Organs such as the liver and intestine	Size
	Shape
	Presence of tenderness
	Presence or absence of masses
	Vibration of voice sounds (lung)

Area of Body Examined	Criteria Measured by Palpation
Glands such as the thyroid and lymph	Swelling Symmetry Mobility
Blood vessels such as the carotid or femoral artery	Pulse amplitude Elasticity Pulse rate Pulse rhythm
Muscles	Size Shape Tone Presence of tenderness Presence of spasm or rigidity
Bones	Symmetry Shape Presence of deformity Presence of tenderness

Percussion

Percussion is striking the body's surface with a finger to produce sound and vibration that determine the location, size, and density of underlying structures to verify abnormalities assessed by palpation and auscultation.

- Table 3 describes the five basic percussion sounds, the sites at which they are normally heard, and the sound characteristics to assess.
- Knowledge of the normal densities of various organs allows the examiner to locate an organ or mass and determine its size by feeling its boundaries.
- Direct method of percussion:
  The body is struck directly with one or two fingertips.
- Indirect method of percussion:
  The middle finger of the nondominant hand (pleximeter) is placed firmly against the body surface (Fig. 4).
  The tip of the middle finger of the dominant hand (plexor) strikes the base of the distal joint of the pleximeter.
  The blow should be struck with a quick, sharp stroke, with the forearm stationary and the wrist relaxed.

Table 3   Sounds produced by percussion

Percussion Sound	Intensity	Pitch	Duration	Quality	Anatomic Location Where Examiner Hears Sounds
Tympany	Loud	High	Moderate	Drumlike	Air-enclosed space, gastric air bubble, puffed-out cheek
Resonance	Moderate to loud	Low	Long	Hollow	Normal lung
Hyperresonance	Very loud	Very low	Longer than resonance	Booming	Emphysematous lung
Dullness	Soft to moderate	High	Moderate	Thudlike	Liver
Flatness	Soft	High	Short	Flat	Muscle

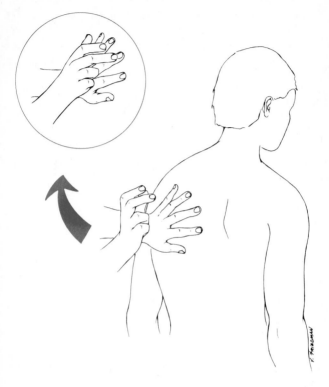

Fig. 4
Technique for applying indirect percussion.

- Apply the same force at each area of the body to make an accurate comparison of sounds produced by percussion.

Auscultation

Auscultation is listening to sounds created in body organs to detect variations from normal.
- Because abnormal sounds can be recognized only in comparison with normal variations, the nurse should learn the types of sounds normally heard at different sites.
- Be sure earpieces of stethoscope fit snugly and comfortably,

with binaurals angled and earpieces following the contour of the ear canal (most persons wear earpieces pointed toward the face).
- Rubber or plastic tubing of stethoscope should be flexible and 30 to 40 cm (12 to 18 inches) in length.
- The examiner with a hearing disorder should use a stethoscope with greater amplification or ask colleagues to validate findings.
- The stethoscope bell is best for low-pitched sounds such as abnormal heart and vascular sounds, and the diaphragm is best for high-pitched sounds such as bowel, lung, and normal heart sounds.
- All sounds have four characteristics that should be assessed:
  Pitch is the measurement of sound frequency, ranging from high to low.
  Loudness is the amplitude of a sound wave, ranging from soft to loud.
  Quality is a characteristic that distinguishes sounds of similar frequency and loudness, described by terms such as blowing, swishing, and gurgling.
  Duration is the length of time a sound lasts as a continuous sound, ranging from short to medium to long.
- With auscultation at any site, the nurse should consider the origin and cause of the sound, the exact site at which it is heard best, and the normal qualities of the sound to assess deviations from normal.

Preparation for the Examination

Preparation should be made for all aspects of the physical assessment, including the environment and the client, to ensure complete and accurate findings. The environment should be suitable for all phases of the examination, with all equipment and supplies readily available. Physical and psychologic preparation of the client helps ensure that the examination proceeds smoothly, without interruption, and without stress for either the client or the nurse.

Preparation of Environment

- Conduct the examination in a well-equipped room if possible. If you are examining the client in a semiprivate hospital room, close the room curtains or dividers to ensure privacy. In the home use the client's bedroom.
- Be sure lighting is adequate.
- A sound-proofed room is ideal; minimize any extraneous sounds or noise.
- Take precautions to prevent interruptions from other health care workers during the examination.
- If an examination table is used, ensure client comfort by offering a small pillow.
    Raise the head of the table about 30 degrees when the client is supine.
    Help the client move onto and off the table, if necessary.
    Do not leave confused, combative, or uncooperative clients unattended on the examining table.
- With infants and older adults, make sure the room is sufficiently warm to maintain comfort.

Preparation of Equipment

- Have all equipment ready before the examination begins to avoid prolonging the examination.

- Use your hands or warm water to warm any equipment that will touch the client.
- Be sure all equipment is functioning properly. Have spare batteries and light bulbs available for the otoscope and ophthalmoscope.
- The following box lists equipment and supplies typically

Equipment and Supplies for Physical Assessment

Blood pressure cuff
Cotton-tipped applicators
Disposable pads
Drapes
Eye chart, such as a Snellen chart
Flashlight and spotlight
Forms, such as for a physical or a laboratory analysis
Gloves (sterile or clean)
Gown for client
Lubricant
Ophthalmoscope
Otoscope
Papanicolaou smear slides
Paper towels
Percussion hammer
Safety pins
Scale with height measurement rod
Specimen containers and microscope slides
Sphygmomanometer
Stethoscope
Swabs or sponge forceps
Tape measure
Thermometer
Tissues
Tongue depressor
Tuning fork
Vaginal speculum
Wristwatch with second hand

needed by examiners for physical assessment (special equipment for special procedures is listed in later chapters).

Physical Preparation of Client

- Ensure the client's physical comfort before starting the examination. Ask the client to empty bladder or bowel if needed, and collect urine and fecal specimens at this time.
- Be sure the client is dressed and draped properly.

  Hospitalized clients generally can wear a simple gown.

  Outpatients can change into a linen or disposable gown.

  To avoid embarrassment, allow the client to change in privacy.
- If the client is uncomfortable with low room temperatures or drafts, provide a blanket as needed.
- Periodically ask whether the client is comfortable.

  Older clients are more likely to become chilled.

  Offering a drink of water, tissue, or pillow may help the client relax.
- Take special care when positioning the client during the examination.

  If the client has limited strength, provide assistance in assuming a position.

  Because many positions are uncomfortable or embarrassing, examiners should not keep the client in these positions longer than necessary.

  Adjust draping during positioning to be sure the body part being examined is accessible but no part is unnecessarily exposed.

  When alternative positions can be used for a particular examination, choose the position best suited for weakened clients.

  With older adults, position the client to avoid looking into the source of light, which can cause discomfort from the light's glare.
- Table 4 describes the standard examination positions for different parts of the physical assessment.

Table 4   Positions for examination

Position	Areas Assessed	Rationale	Limitations
Sitting	Head and neck, back, posterior thorax and lungs, anterior thorax and lungs, breasts, axilla, heart, vital signs, and upper extremities	Sitting upright provides full expansion of lungs and provides better visualization of symmetry of upper body parts	Client who is physically weakened may be unable to sit; use supine position with head of bed elevated instead
Supine	Head and neck, anterior thorax and lungs, breasts, axilla, heart, abdomen, extremities, pulses	Most normally relaxed position; prevents contracture of abdominal muscles; provides easy access to pulse sites	If client becomes short of breath easily, examiner may need to raise head of bed
Dorsal recumbent	Head and neck, anterior thorax and lungs, breasts, axilla, heart	Certain clients with painful disorders are more comfortable with knees flexed	Not used for abdominal assessment, since position promotes contracture of abdominal muscles

Lithotomy	Female genitalia and genital tract	Provides maximal exposure of genitalia and facilitates insertion of vaginal speculum	Embarrassing and uncomfortable position, thus minimize time client spends in this position; keep client well draped; client with severe arthritis or other joint deformity may be unable to assume position
Sims' position	Rectum	Flexion of hip and knee improves exposure of rectal area	Joint deformities may hinder client's ability to bend hip and knee
Prone	Musculoskeletal	Position used only to assess extension of hip joint	Position intolerable for clients with respiratory difficulties or elderly clients

Psychologic Preparation of Client

Because many clients find a physical examination tiring or stressful or experience anxiety about possible assessment findings, the examiner should psychologically prepare the client before the examination and should attend to the client's emotional state to minimize concerns during the examination.

- Begin by explaining in general terms the purpose of the examination and how it will be performed.
- Tell the client to feel free to ask any questions and provide an opportunity for those questions.
- As you examine each body system, explain the procedure in greater detail.

    Use simple explanations to avoid confusing or frightening the client with unfamiliar terms.

    Use a relaxed tone of voice and facial expression when making explanations, but maintain a professional demeanor.

- If the client is of the opposite sex, it is helpful to have a third person of the client's sex present, particularly when examining the genitalia.
- Monitor the client's emotional responses throughout the examination.

    Observe fear or concern in facial expressions.

    Observe for body movements such as tensing when touched or clutching the drape around the body.

    If the client is overly afraid, anxious, or uncomfortable, postpone the examination until a time when relaxation and cooperation can lead to greater accuracy in the assessment.

General Survey

5

Organization of the Examination

The extent of an examination depends on its purpose. There are clients whose physical condition requires a limited or focused assessment. A client returning from surgery for repair of a fractured leg requires assessment of circulatory and musculoskeletal function rather than a breast examination. When a client is admitted to a hospital or is a first-time visitor to a clinic, a complete examination is usually performed.

The assessment follows certain priorities when a client is ill or has specific symptoms. Body systems most at risk should be examined first in such cases; noncritical parts of the examination can be deferred until the client can tolerate a more thorough examination. A client who has shortness of breath usually first undergoes a complete thoracic (Chapter 17) and cardiac (Chapter 18) assessment. A more extensive examination can wait until the client's fatigue is relieved.

Complete physical assessments generally should be performed after the nursing history is taken. Information from the history can focus the examiner's attention on specific body parts or systems so that assessment data supplement, confirm, or refute data from the history. The organization of the examination usually follows a head-to-toe approach to ensure that all body systems are reviewed.

Tips for keeping an examination organized include the following:

1. Compare both sides of the body for symmetry. A degree of asymmetry is normal (for example, the biceps muscle of the dominant arm may be more developed than the same muscle in the nondominant arm).

2. Perform painful assessment procedures near the end of the examination.

3. If a client becomes fatigued, offer rest periods between assessments.

4. Record findings in specific anatomic and scientific terms so that any professional can interpret the results of the examination.
5. Use common and accepted medical abbreviations to keep notes brief and concise.
6. Record quick notes during the examination to avoid keeping the client waiting.
7. Complete all observations after the examination. Use an assessment form organized in the same sequence as the examination.

General Survey

The nurse begins an examination by observing the client's general appearance and behavior and by measuring vital signs (Part II) and height and weight. At times the nurse also makes anthropometric measurements, including head, chest, or abdominal circumference of infants.

Rationale

The general survey provides information about characteristics of an illness, a client's hygiene and body image, recent changes in weight that may reveal presence of disease, and the client's developmental status.

Special Equipment

- Weighing scale (standing or bed) with height measuring attachment
- Thermometer
- Sphygmomanometer
- Stethoscope

Client Preparation

- Conduct the general survey with the client sitting or standing. An experienced nurse can do this almost automatically before beginning the physical assessment.
- Ask the client to remove shoes and any heavy outer clothing before you measure height and weight.
- When weighing a hospitalized client, always weigh at the same time of day, with the same scale, and with the client wearing the same clothing.

History

- Ask the client for current height and weight.
- Ask whether the client has had a recent change in weight or appetite.
- Ask the client's reason for seeking health care.
- Ask what the client's primary health problems are.

Assessment Techniques

Review the client's general appearance and behavior.

- Sex and race. The client's sex affects the type of examination performed and the manner in which assessments are made. Different physical features are related to sex and age. Certain illnesses are more likely to affect a specific sex or race.
- Signs of distress. There may be obvious signs or symptoms indicating a problem such as pain or difficulty breathing.
- Body type. Note if client appears trim and muscular, obese, or excessively thin. Body type reflects level of health, age, and life-style.
- Posture. Normal standing posture is an upright stance with parallel alignment of hips and shoulders. Normal sitting involves some rounding of the shoulders. Note whether the client has a slumped, erect, or bent posture. Posture may reflect mood or presence of pain.
- Gait. Observe the client walk into the room or along the bedside (if ambulatory). Note whether movements are coordinated or uncoordinated. A person normally walks with the arms swinging freely at the sides and with the head and face leading the body.
- Body movements. Observe whether movements are purposeful, there are tremors involving the extremities, and any body parts are immobile.
- Age. Normal physical characteristics vary according to a client's age. The ability to participate in an examination is also influenced by age.
- Hygiene and grooming. Note the client's level of cleanliness by observing the appearance of the hair, skin, and fingernails. Note whether the client's clothes are clean. A person's grooming may be affected by degree of illness, as well as the type of activities performed just before the examination.
- Dress. A person's culture, life-style, socioeconomic level, and personal preference affect the type of clothes worn. Note

whether the type of clothing worn is appropriate for temperature and weather conditions. Depressed or mentally ill persons may be unable to choose proper clothing. Elderly people may wear extra clothing because of their sensitivity to cold.

- Body odor. An unpleasant body odor may simply be the result of physical exercise or may be caused by poor hygiene. Poor oral hygiene may result in bad breath.
- Mood and affect. Affect is a person's feelings as they appear to others. A person's mood or emotional state is expressed verbally and nonverbally. Observe whether the client's mood is appropriate for the situation.
- Speech. Normal speech is understandable and moderately paced and shows an association with the person's thoughts. Note whether the client talks rapidly or slowly. An abnormal pace may be caused by emotions or neurologic impairment.

Measurement of Height and Weight

- Weigh the client using a standing scale. Use a stretcher scale for clients who are unable to bear weight. Use a table scale for infants; weigh an infant unclothed and protect the infant from falling from the scale basket.
- With the client standing erect on a scale, raise the metal rod attached to the scale up and over the client's head. The rod should be placed level horizontally at a 90-degree angle to the measuring stick. Height is measured in inches or centimeters.

Measure the Client's Vital Signs

- See Part II for guidelines. Most nurses prefer measuring vital signs before assessing body systems because positioning or moving the client may interfere with accurate measurements.

Normal findings

Height-weight correlations (Appendix A) and growth tables indicate average normal findings for adults and children at different developmental levels.

Deviations from normal

A discrepancy between the client's perception of height and weight and the actual measurements may indicate a potential body image problem.

Recent weight gains or losses may indicate serious disease. A weight gain of up to 5 pounds (2.3 kg) in a day may indicate a fluid retention problem.

Nurse alert

In an adult, significant variations in height and weight from the normal values may indicate nutritional or other serious health problems. In children, significant deviations from normal may also indicate hormonal disturbances, but the examiner should also consider that height and weight extremes may be a result of hereditary factors.

Pediatric considerations

An infant can be measured by placing the child supine on a hard, flat surface, with the knees extended and the soles supported upright and measuring from the soles of the feet to the vertex of the head.

If a child is below minimum height on the standing scale, position the child against a wall, place a book on top of the child's head perpendicular to the wall, mark the wall at the point of contact, and measure the distance between the floor and the mark on the wall.

Gerontologic considerations

Older adults may have a decrease in height as a result of osteoporosis and kyphosis.

Anthropometric Measurements

In addition to measurements of height and weight, measurements of circumference of the arm, chest, and head of an infant can indicate nutritional status and provide data about growth and development.

Rationale

Measuring an infant's head circumference allows an estimation of brain growth. Measures of arm circumference indicate musculature development and protein and caloric intake.

Special equipment

Tape measures.

Assessment techniques

Assessment	Normal Findings

Measure the infant's head circumference:
Have the child lie supine.

Place measuring tape at greatest circumference anteriorly over lower forehead above supraorbital ridges and posteriorly over occipital bone (Fig. 5).

Normal head circumference at birth ranges from 12.4 to 14.8 inches (31 to 37 cm).

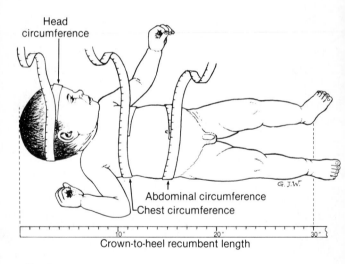

Fig. 5
Measuring infant's head, chest, and abdominal circumference.
(From Wong DL and Whaley LF: Clinical handbook of pediatric nursing, ed 2, St. Louis, 1986, The CV Mosby Co.

Assessment	Normal Findings
Measure the infant's chest circumference:	
Have the child lie supine. Measure chest diameter at the infant's nipple line.	At birth, head circumference exceeds chest circumference by 1 inch.
	In infants (1 to 2 years of age) head circumference equals chest circumference.
	In toddlers (3 to 4 years of age) head circumference is 2 to 4 inches smaller than chest circumference.
Measure the infant's abdominal circumference:	The abdomen in a normal infant is cylindric.
Have the child lie supine. Measure the infant's abdominal circumference at the umbilicus.	

Deviations from Normal

Large infant head size may indicate congenital anomalies or hydrocephalus.

Small infant head size may indicate underdevelopment.

MEASUREMENT OF VITAL SIGNS

II

Vital signs are measured to determine a client's usual state of health (baseline data) or to determine a client's response to physiologic or psychologic stress or to medical or nursing therapies. Vital signs are measured as a part of a complete physical assessment but may be measured separately as a quick way to review the client's condition or identify a problem.

Guidelines for Incorporating Vital Signs in Nursing Practice

- Know the client's normal range of vital signs and compare measurements with these values.
- Know the client's medical history and any medications or therapies being received that may affect vital signs.
- Control environmental factors that influence vital signs.
- Decide the frequency of vital sign assessment on the basis of the client's condition.
- Be sure equipment used in measurement is appropriate and functional.
- Use an organized, systematic method to measure vital signs.
- Verify significant changes in vital signs and notify the physician immediately of abnormal values.
- Know the clinical implications of vital sign abnormalities to initiate specific interventions as needed.

The box describes when vital signs generally should be measured.

When to Take Vital Signs

On the client's admission to hospital or health care facility.

In a hospital on a routine frequency according to a physician's orders or hospital policy.

Before and after any surgical procedure.

Before and after any invasive diagnostic procedure.

Before and after administration of medications that affect cardiovascular, respiratory, and temperature control functions.

When the client's general physical condition changes (as with increased intensity of pain or onset of confusion).

Before and after nursing interventions that may influence any one of the vital signs (for example, before ambulation of a client previously restricted to bed rest or before a client performs range-of-motion exercises).

Whenever the client reports to the nurse any nonspecific symptoms of physical distress such as "feeling funny or different."

Body Temperature 6

Normal Body Temperature

The average normal adult body temperature is 98.6° F (37° C) ± 1° F. Fig. 6 shows the range of normal temperatures for healthy adults under various conditions.

Physiology of Body Temperature

- Heat is normally produced in the body in four ways:

    Basal metabolism constitutes 55% to 60% of a person's total metabolic rate, or the amount of energy used by the body at any time.

    Muscular activity, including shivering, raises the metabolic rate and therefore heat production.

    Thyroid hormone secretion increases basal metabolism.

    Stimulation of the sympathetic nervous system by epinephrine and norepinephrine increases heat production in the body.

- Heat is lost from the body through four mechanisms. Impairment of these mechanisms can result in fever.

    Heat is lost by radiation of infrared rays from the skin. Radiation is greater when blood vessels are dilated.

    Heat is lost by conduction to objects touching the body or to water cooler than body temperature.

    Heat is lost as heated air along the skin's surface passes to cooler air by convection currents.

    Heat is lost by the evaporative effect of sweating.

- The body normally maintains a balance between heat production and heat loss through the mechanisms of temperature control:

    The hypothalamus acts as a thermostat, sensing minor changes in body temperature and activating heat loss or pro-

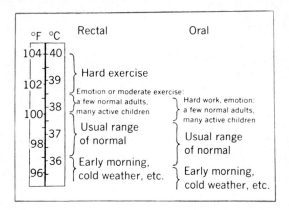

Fig. 6

Ranges in rectal and oral temperatures found in normal persons.

(From Mountcastle VB: Medical physiology, vol 2, St Louis, 1980, The CV Mosby Co.)

duction to keep the core temperature in a safe physiologic range.

Behavioral regulation involves the voluntary acts, such as adding clothing or moving to a warmer or cooler place, that maintain a comfortable body temperature.

The skin insulates the body against heat loss, promotes heat loss by radiating heat from the blood to the air, and contains receptors to sense surface temperatures so that the hypothalamus initiates thermoregulation reflexes.

Sweat glands when stimulated release moisture that evaporates to facilitate heat loss.

Rationale

In addition to being able to correctly determine a client's body temperature, the nurse should understand the significance of findings to effectively assess the client's health status and intervene if problems are indicated. This understanding includes the normal range of body temperature and the factors that can affect the client's temperature, the physiology of heat production and loss, the mechanisms of temperature control, and the significance of fever.

Factors Affecting Body Temperature

Factor	Effect
Age	The neonate's temperature normally ranges from 96° F to 99.5° F (35.5° C to 37.5° C).
	Temperature regulation is labile until puberty.
	With old age the normal range commonly lowers, with 96.8° F (36° C) normal for some elderly clients.
Exercise	Prolonged strenuous exercise can temporarily raise body temperatures as high as 105° F (41° C).
Diurnal variations	The body temperature normally is at its lowest between 1 AM and 4 AM.
	Temperature usually peaks between 4 PM and 7 PM on the average.
	Each client has a different temperature pattern.
Stress	Physical or emotional stress, such as anxiety related to physical assessment, may raise body temperature.
Environment	Environmental temperature extremes can raise or lower the body temperature, depending on extent of exposure, air humidity, and presence of convection currents.

Fever

- A fever is a body temperature of more than 100.4° F (38° C) in resting conditions.
- A fever results from an alteration in the hypothalamus set point by pyrogens, which raise the body temperature.
- Physiologic responses to fever include the following:
  Production and conservation of heat through vasoconstriction, shivering, and piloerection.
  Increased metabolism and oxygen consumption.
  Increased heart and respiratory rates.

Risks of dehydration.

Restlessness and disorientation if oxygen needs are not met.

Convulsions in children with high fevers.

- Fever is an important defense mechanism that may help activate the body's immune system by stimulating release of interleukin-1, which stimulates antibody production.

Nursing Diagnosis

- Assessment data may reveal the following nursing diagnoses related to fever:

    Pain related to fever

    Hyperthermia related to infectious process

    Activity intolerance related to reduced energy stores

    Altered nutrition: less than body requirements related to increased metabolism

Nursing Measures for Clients with Fever

- Provide fluids (minimum 3 liters [approximately 12 cups] per day if cardiac and renal function are normal).
- Give tepid bath to reduce body surface temperature.
- Meet oral hygiene needs to prevent drying of mucous membranes.
- Reduce external body covering, but do not induce chills.
- Keep clothing and bedding dry.
- Provide well-balanced meals.
- Reduce exhaustive activities.
- Provide supplemental oxygen as needed.
- Monitor pulse and respiration.
- Control temperature of the environment without causing chills.

Special Equipment

The following equipment is used in assessing body temperature:

    Mercury in glass thermometers, including oral, stubby (for any site), and rectal types

    Electronic thermometers (with oral or rectal disposable plastic probe covers)

    Disposable single-use thermometers—may be used for oral temperatures or can be applied to the skin

    Soft tissue

Lubricant (rectal measurements only)
Sink with running water
Storage container with disinfectant (glass thermometers)
Disposable glove

Preparation

Select the most appropriate measurement site.

Oral

Advantages	Contraindications
Most accessible More comfortable Reading is accurate	Risk of injury to client, client unable to hold thermometer in mouth, risk of client biting down, such as with infant or small child, confusion, unconsciousness, after oral surgery, mouth or facial trauma, pain in mouth, breathing only through mouth, history of convulsions, shaking chill, or client receiving oxygen therapy

Rectal

Advantages	Contraindications
Argued as most reliable when oral cannot be taken Used with infants	Rectal surgery or disorder such as tumor or hemorrhoids; clients who cannot be positioned properly such as those in traction

Axillary

Advantages	Contraindications
Least risk of injury Used with newborn	Used only when oral or rectal site cannot be used

Client Preparation

- Position the client properly and if necessary explain the procedure and its purpose.

- Have all equipment and supplies ready to avoid interrupting the procedure.
- Wash hands, using aseptic technique.
- For oral measurements, wait 30 minutes after the ingestion of any hot or cold foods or liquids or after smoking.
- Apply disposable glove to dominant hand.

Assessment Techniques—Objective Data
Oral measurement

- Hold the thermometer by color-coded end or top of stem.
- Rinse in cold water, if stored in disinfectant (mercury thermometer).
- Wipe the thermometer with tissue from bulb to end with a rotary motion and dispose of the tissue (mercury thermometer).
- For an electronic thermometer add a disposable plastic probe cover over the thermometer.
- Read the mercury level; if more than 96° F (35.5° C), shake down with sharp wrist flick (mercury thermometer).
- Place the thermometer in sublingual pocket, lateral to center of lower jaw.
- Ask the client to hold the thermometer with lips closed.
- Leave the thermometer in place 2 minutes or according to agency policy (electronic displays in seconds).
- Carefully remove the thermometer and wipe clean again or dispose of plastic probe cover.
- Read the mercury level or digital display.
- Shake the thermometer down again and store properly or return the probe to a storage well.
- Record the temperature.

Rectal measurement

- Rinse, clean, and shake down the rectal thermometer in the same manner as the oral thermometer (mercury thermometer).
- Maintain privacy for the client with drawn curtains or a closed door.
- Keep the client's upper body and lower extremities covered.
- Ask or assist an adult client to assume the Sims position with legs flexed; a child may lie prone.
- Liberally lubricate (water-soluble lubricant) the thermometer's bulb end or the plastic probe 1 to 1½ inches (2.5 to 3.5 cm) for adults or ½ to 1 inch (1.2 to 2.5 cm) for an infant.

- Expose the anus by raising the upper buttock with the nondominant hand; with the infant prone on bed or lap, retract both buttocks with fingers.
- Gently insert the thermometer into the anus in the direction of the umbilicus, 1½ inches (3.5 cm) for adults, ½ inch (1.2 cm) for infants.

    Do not force the thermometer.

    Ask the client to take a deep breath and blow out, inserting the thermometer during deep breathing when the anal sphincter is relaxed.

- If resistance is felt during insertion, withdraw the thermometer immediately.
- Hold the thermometer in place 2 minutes or according to agency policy, holding an infant's legs if necessary (electronic displays in seconds).
- Remove the thermometer and wipe clean in a rotating motion from tip to bulb or dispose of the plastic probe cover on the thermometer.
- Wipe the anal area to remove lubricant or feces.
- Read the mercury level or digital display.
- Help the client into a more comfortable position.
- Wash the thermometer in lukewarm soapy water and rinse in cool water or return the probe to a storage well.
- Dry and shake down the thermometer and return it to the container.
- Remove glove inside out and discard.
- Wash hands.
- Record the temperature, signifying a rectal reading with the letter "R."

Axillary measurement

- Rinse the thermometer in cold water, wipe clean, and shake down (mercury thermometer).
- Assist the client to a sitting or supine position.
- Move clothing or gown from shoulder and arm.
- Insert the thermometer into the center of the axilla, lower the client's arm, and place forearm across the chest.
- Leave the thermometer in place 5 to 10 minutes; with a child, hold arm gently in place (electronic displays in seconds).
- Remove the thermometer and wipe clean.
- Read the mercury level.

- Shake the thermometer down and store in its container or return the probe to a storage well.
- Record temperature, signifying the axillary reading with the letter "A."

Temperature Conversions

To convert from Fahrenheit to centigrade (Celsius):

Subtract 32 from Fahrenheit reading
Multiply the remainder by $\frac{5}{9}$
$C = (F - 32) \times \frac{5}{9}$

To convert centigrade to Fahrenheit:

Multiply the centigrade reading by $\frac{9}{5}$
Add 32 to the product
$F = (\frac{9}{5} \times C) + 32$

Client Teaching

All clients should know how to safely and accurately measure body temperature for health promotion purposes. It is particularly important to teach clients with febrile illnesses or conditions that increase the risk of infection and parents of children who are unable to measure their own temperature.

Pulse

7

Anatomy and Physiology

- Blood flows through the body in a continuous circuit as the heart ejects blood intermittently into the arterial system.
- With each ventricular contraction, approximately 60 to 70 ml of blood enters the aorta, distending the aortic walls and creating the pulse wave.
- Cardiac output is the volume of blood pumped by the heart in 1 minute, normally averaging about 5000 ml.
- Cardiac output is the product of ventricular stroke volume and heart rate. If either component is reduced, the other attempts to compensate to maintain a stable cardiac output.

Rationale

Pulse assessment provides data about the integrity of the cardio-vascular system. The nurse routinely assesses the rate, rhythm, strength, elasticity, and equality of pulses. An abnormally slow, rapid, or irregular pulse may indicate a problem in circulatory regulation. A cardiac dysrhythmia, or abnormal rhythm, may threaten the heart's ability to function properly. The strength of a pulse reflects the volume of blood ejected with each heart contraction. Assessment of arterial elasticity may reveal conditions, such as arteriosclerosis, that change the quality of arterial walls. Comparing pulses on both sides of the body for equality may reveal variations such as local interruptions to blood flow caused by a blood clot.

Pulse Assessment
Preparation

Select the appropriate pulse site(s).

Radial pulse

Advantages	Disadvantages
Most accessible pulse	Dressings, casts, and other encumbrances may block site
Easily palpated	Less accurate with infants and young children

Apical pulse

Advantages	Disadvantages
Used when radial pulse site is inaccessible	Requires auscultation of heart sounds
Most accurate for assessing heart function in cases of cardiac disease	
Used to confirm abnormalities detected in radial pulse	
Best site to assess infant's or young child's heart rate	

Carotid pulse

Advantages	Disadvantages
Easily accessible pulse	None
Best for finding pulse quickly when client's condition deteriorates	

Other sites

Assessment of other peripheral pulse sites (Chapter 18), such as the brachial or femoral pulse sites, is performed during a complete physical examination, when surgery or treatment impairs blood flow to a body part, or when it is necessary to assess indications of impaired peripheral blood flow.

Special Equipment

The following equipment is used in assessing the pulse:
   A watch with second hand or digital display

Client Preparation

- Position the client supine with a forearm across the lower chest or at the side of the body. If the client is seated, bend the elbow 90 degrees and support the lower arm on the chair or on your arm.
- If the client has been active, wait 5 to 10 minutes before assessing the pulse.
- Explain the purpose and method of the procedure to the client.

History

- Determine whether the client is receiving any medications that might affect heart rate or contraction.
- Consider factors involving the client that might affect pulse rate (Table 5).

Table 5   Factors that influence pulse rate

Factor	Effect
Exercise	Short-term effect—increased rate
	Long-term effect—strengthens heart muscle, resulting in lower-than-normal rate at rest and a quicker return to resting rate after exercise
Fever, heat	Increases rate
Acute pain, anxiety	Sympathetic stimulation—increases rate
Unrelieved, severe pain	Parasympathetic stimulation—slows rate
Medications	
Digitalis	Slows rate
Atropine	Increases rate
Hemorrhage (loss of blood)	Increases rate
Postural changes	
Lying	Slows rate
Standing	Increases rate

Assessment Techniques

Procedure	Rationale
Place tips of first two fingers of your hand over groove along radial, or thumb side, of client's inner wrist (Fig. 7).	The fingertips are most sensitive to vibratory sense. Do not palpate with the thumb or you may feel your own pulse accidentally.
Obliterate the pulse initially, then relax pressure so that the pulse is easily palpable.	A pulse is more accurately assessed with moderate pressure. Too much pressure occludes a pulse, and too little pressure prevents the examiner from feeling the pulse with regularity.
Once the pulse can be felt regularly, use the watch's second hand and begin to count the rate, starting with "0," then "1," and so on.	Rate is determined accurately only after assessor is sure that pulse can be palpated. Time interval begins with "0." Count of "1" begins sequence.

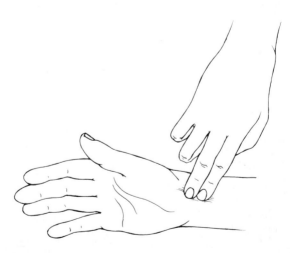

Fig. 7
Radial pulse is detected with pads of fingertips.

Procedure	Rationale
If the pulse is regular, count for 15 seconds and multiply the total number of beats by 4.	A regular rate can be accurately assessed in 15 seconds.
If the pulse is irregular, count 1 full minute.	Ensures accurate count.
Assess rhythm and strength of pulse and elasticity of arterial wall.	Provides complete assessment of pulse character.
Assist client to a comfortable position.	
Record characteristics of pulse in medical record or flow sheets.	Record vital signs immediately.

Pulse Rate

Assessment	Normal Findings
Know the client's baseline heart rate.	Newborn (resting) 100 to 180 beats/min Infant (resting) 80 to 150 beats/min Child 2 to 10 years of age 70 to 110 beats/min Adolescent 11 years of age to adult 55 to 90 beats/min
Once the pulse is felt regularly, count rate for 15 seconds and multiply total by four if the rate is regular.	
If pulse is irregular, count for 1 full minute.	
Compare assessed rate with baseline rate.	
Assess apical pulse if heart rate is outside normal range (Chapter 18).	Radial and apical pulse rates should be equal.

Assessment	Normal Findings
Optionally, assess baseline measurements with client sitting, standing, or lying; maintain consistency of position when making comparisons.	

Deviations from Normal

Tachycardia (rate about 100 beats/min)
Bradycardia (rate less than 55 beats/min)

Pulse Rhythm

Assessment	Normal Findings
Note whether the heartbeats occur successively at regular intervals.	Regardless of pulse rate or strength, the rhythm is normally regular.
If irregular rhythm (dysrhythmia) is detected in the client, assess the regularity of its occurrence.	
The physician may order an electrocardiogram to confirm a dysrhythmia.	
If cardiac dysrhythmia is present, assess the client's apical pulse in conjunction with radial pulse to detect any pulse deficit.	

Deviations from Normal

Any dysrhythmia should be reported to the physician. (See p. 157 for types of dysrhythmia.)
In a pulse deficit the radial pulse is usually slower than the apical pulse.

Pulse Strength

Assessment	Normal Findings
Assess pulse strength while measuring rate and observing rhythm. Pulse strength is a subjective determination, based on practice and experience.	Pulse strength remains consistent with each beat. Normal pulse is full, easily palpated, and not easily obliterated by assessor's fingers.

Deviations from Normal

A bounding pulse is easy to palpate and difficult to obliterate.

A weak pulse is thready in character, often rapid, difficult to palpate, and easy to lose.

See p. 163 for a pulse classification system.

Arterial Elasticity

Assessment	Normal Findings
Gently palpate the artery's walls to determine their characteristics.	Artery is straight, smooth, round, and elastic.

Deviations from Normal

Artery walls harden, become cordlike, and may be tortuous in conditions such as arteriosclerosis.

Pulse Equality Assessment

Assessment	Normal Findings
Compare pulses on both sides of the peripheral vascular system to determine equality in all characteristics.	All pulse characteristics are similar on both sides.

Deviations from Normal

Significant variations between the two sides may indicate an abnormal condition such as blood flow interrupted by a clot or thrombus.

Nursing Diagnosis

- Assessment data may help reveal the following nursing diagnoses:

    Decreased cardiac output related to cardiac dysrhythmias

    Altered peripheral tissue perfusion related to arterial obstruction

Client Teaching

Clients receiving medications for heart diseases should learn to measure pulse to detect alterations in rate or rhythm that may indicate side effects of the medications or worsening of their conditions.

Clients involved in exercise training learn to palpate either their radial or carotid arteries. Caution clients against palpating both carotid arteries simultaneously, which can reduce blood flow to the brain.

Respiration

8

Anatomy and Physiology

- Respiration involves four interrelated processes:

   Ventilation—movement of air into and out of the lungs

   Conduction—movement of air through lung airways

   Diffusion—movement of O_2 and CO_2 between alveoli and red blood cells

   Perfusion—distribution of blood flow through pulmonary capillaries

- Respiration is involuntarily controlled by the respiratory center in the brainstem.

   Ventilation is regulated according to arterial blood levels of CO_2, O_2, and pH; the P_{CO_2} level is the most important factor.

   An elevated P_{CO_2} level leads to increased rate and depth of ventilation.

   A lowered O_2 level (hypoxia—as occurs in emphysema and bronchitis) leads to increased rate and depth of ventilation.

- The mechanics of breathing involve the muscles of inspiration and expiration.

   In inspiration, impulses from the respiratory center by means of the phrenic nerve to the diaphragm stimulate diaphragmatic contraction.

   With diaphragm contraction, abdominal organs move downward and forward and the ribs upward and outward to facilitate lung expansion.

   In expiration, a relatively passive process, the lung, chest wall, and diaphragm return to the relaxed position.

   Passive breathing is more diaphragmatic; active or costal breathing involves more rib movement and active work of intercostal and accessory muscles.

- The character of ventilation is affected by conditions that impair respiratory processes.

   Clients with a reduced red blood cell count ventilate at a faster rate to increase oxygen delivery.

Clients with chest wall pain may voluntarily splint or inhibit ventilatory movement and breathe less deeply.

See also the assessment of the thorax, p. 137.

Rationale

Assessment of the processes of external respiration focuses on the characteristics of ventilation; assessment of internal respiration—the exchange of oxygen and carbon dioxide at the cellular level—depends on laboratory tests. Assessment includes the rate, depth, and rhythm of ventilatory movements and observation of general respiratory character.

Respiration Assessment
Special Equipment

A watch with second hand or digital display

Client Preparation

- Allow the client to assume a comfortable position, preferably sitting or lying with the head of the bed elevated 45 to 60 degrees.
- If the client has been active, wait 5 to 10 minutes before assessing respirations.

History

- Assess for factors that normally influence character of respirations (Table 6).

Assessment Techniques

Procedure	Rationale
Draw curtain around client's bed or close room door. Be sure client's chest is visible. Adjust bed linen or gown.	Provides for client's privacy. Provides for visualization of chest for thorough assessment.
Have client's arm placed in a relaxed position across abdomen or lower chest (alternative—place your hand directly over client's upper abdomen).	This position is used during assessment of the pulse. The client's (or nurse's) hand will rise and fall during the respiratory cycle.

Table 6   Factors that influence respiration

Factor	Effect
Exercise	Increases rate and depth. More active than passive breathing.
Anxiety, fear	Increases rate and depth.
Self-consciousness (awareness of respiratory assessment)	Client may consciously alter rate and depth.
Disease or illness	May increase or decrease rate and depth or affect rhythm.
Medication, therapy	May increase or decrease rate and depth or affect rhythm. CNS depressants reduce rate and depth.
Fever	Increases rate.
Cigarette smoking	Long-term effects may include increased rate.
Body position	In slumped or stooped position, ventilation is often impaired, with reduced rate.
Sex	Men have greater lung vital capacity than women.
Age	With growth from infancy to adulthood, lung vital capacity increases; with old age, lung elasticity and depth of respiration decrease.

Procedure	Rationale
Observe a complete respiratory cycle.	One respiration consists of one inspiration and one expiration.
In an adult count respirations for 30 seconds and multiply by 2. In an infant or young child count respirations for 1 full minute.	The respiratory rate is equivalent to the number of respirations per minute. Young infants and children breathe in an irregular rhythm.

Procedure	Rationale
If an adult's respirations are irregular in rhythm or abnormally slow or fast, count 1 full minute.	Accurate interpretation requires assessment for at least 1 minute.
While counting, note depth and rhythm of respirations. Depth is shallow, normal, or deep; rhythm is normal or one of the altered patterns (see Table 6).	The character of ventilatory movements may reveal specific alterations or disease states.
Record results in a chart form or flow sheet.	Record vital signs immediately to ensure accuracy.

Respiration rate

Assessment	Normal Findings
Count number of respirations per minute.	Infant: 30 to 60 breaths/min
2 years of age: 20 to 30 breaths/min
6 years of age: 18 to 24 breaths/min
12 years of age: 17 to 21 breaths/min
Adult: 12 to 20 breaths/min
Older adult: the number of respirations per minute is gradually increasing

Deviations from Normal

Depressed or elevated rate outside normal range without influencing factor.
See Table 7 for alterations.

Table 7   Alterations in respirations

Terminology	Description
Bradypnea	An abnormally slow but regular rate of breathing.
Tachypnea	An abnormally rapid but regular rate of breathing.
Hyperpnea	Increased depth and rate of respirations. Occurs normally with exercise.
Apnea	A cessation of respirations. Persistent cessation is called respiratory arrest.
Hyperventilation	Rate of ventilation exceeds normal metabolic requirements for exchange of respiratory gases. The rate and depth of respirations increase. There is an excess intake of oxygen and blowing off of carbon dioxide.
Hypoventilation	The volume of air entering the lungs is insufficient for the body's metabolic needs. The respiratory rate is below normal, and depth of ventilation is depressed.
Cheyne-Stokes	Irregular respiratory rhythm characterized by alternating periods of apnea and hyperventilation. The respiratory cycle begins with slow shallow breaths that gradually increase to abnormal depth and rapidity. Breathing gradually slows and becomes shallower, climaxing in a 10- to 20-second period of apnea before respiration resumes.
Kussmaul	Abnormally deep respirations with a regular rhythm, similar to hyperventilation. Characteristic in clients with diabetic ketoacidosis.
Dyspnea	Difficulty in breathing, characterized by an increased effort to inhale and exhale air. The person actively uses intercostal and accessory muscles to breathe.

Respiration depth

Assessment	Normal Findings
Observe chest wall movement. Depth assessment is generally a subjective evaluation based on practice and experience. Optionally, measure chest wall excursion, a more objective measure (see Chapter 17).	Normal tidal breath is about 500 cc of air. Diaphragm moves about ½ inch (1.2 cm). Ribs retract about 1 to 2 inches (2.5 to 5 cm).

Deviations from Normal

With shallow breathing, ventilatory movement is almost imperceptible.

With deep breathing, the lungs expand fully and exhalation is full and often audible.

See Table 6 for alterations.

Respiration rhythm

Assessment	Normal Findings
Note whether respirations occur successively at regular intervals.	Respirations occur in regular, uninterrupted rhythm.
If irregular rhythm is observed, assess the regularity of its occurrence.	Infants normally breathe less regularly (for example, sudden increases in rate).
Report any irregular rhythm to the physician.	

Deviations from Normal

Any irregular rhythm may indicate illness or a respiratory problem.
See Table 6 for alterations.

General respiratory character

Assessment	Normal Findings
Observe client's skin and nail bed color.	With adequate respiration and oxygenation, skin color is normal.
Observe level of consciousness.	With proper oxygenation client should be alert and oriented unless other alterations are present.
Observe whether client breathes with effort.	
Listen for any audible breathing sounds.	Normal restful breathing is effortless.
See p. 143 for auscultation of lung sounds.	Breathing is not normally audible without a stethoscope.

Deviations from Normal

Bluish or cyanotic color of nail beds, lips, or skin may indicate reduced arterial oxygen.

Restlessness or anxiety may result from reduced oxygenation.

Dyspnea (increased breathing effort) may indicate a respiratory problem.

Breathing sounds heard without a stethoscope include stridor, which may indicate an obstructed air flow caused by inflammation or a stricture.

See Fig. 8 for alterations.

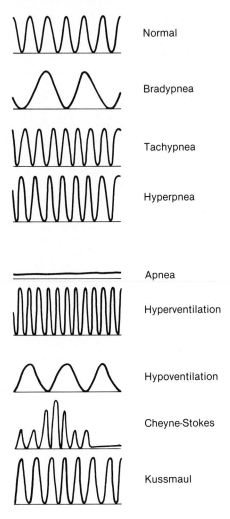

Normal

Bradypnea

Tachypnea

Hyperpnea

Apnea

Hyperventilation

Hypoventilation

Cheyne-Stokes

Kussmaul

Fig. 8
Diagrammatic representations of variations in respiration.

Nursing Diagnoses

■ Assessment data may reveal the following nursing diagnoses:
    Ineffective airway clearance related to thickened secretions or fatigue
    Ineffective breathing pattern related to pain or anxiety
    Impaired gas exchange related to infectious process

Client Teaching

Clients with preexisting respiratory disease should be taught preventive measures for avoiding respiratory infections. Special breathing exercises may be necessary for clients with chronic lung disease.

Educate clients about the association of cigarette smoking with pulmonary disease.

Blood Pressure

9

Anatomy and Physiology

- Blood pressure is the force exerted by the blood against the arterial wall.

    Systolic pressure is the maximum pressure during systole as the left ventricle pumps blood into the aorta.

    Diastolic pressure is the minimum pressure as the ventricles relax.

    The pulse pressure is the difference between systolic and diastolic pressures.

- Blood pressure reflects the relationship among cardiac output, peripheral vascular resistance, blood volume, blood viscosity, and arterial elasticity.

    Each of these factors significantly affects the others.

    Physiologic compensatory mechanisms normally maintain a balance of factors to compensate for changes in any one variable.

- Blood pressure is a product of cardiac output and peripheral vascular resistance.

    Increased cardiac output raises the blood pressure; decreased output lowers it.

    Increased vascular resistance raises the blood pressure; decreased resistance lowers it.

Rationale

Because blood pressure is influenced by many hemodynamic variables, assessment of a client's blood pressure provides important data about a client's hemodynamic status and overall health condition. The following material shows hemodynamic variables that may be associated with increased or decreased blood pressure.

Variables Associated with Increased Blood Pressure	Variables Associated with Decreased Blood Pressure
Increased cardiac output	Decreased cardiac output
Increased peripheral vascular resistance	Decreased peripheral vascular resistance
Increased blood volume	Decreased blood volume
Increased blood viscosity	Decreased blood viscosity
Decreased arterial elasticity	Increased arterial elasticity

Blood Pressure Assessment
Special Equipment

Stethoscope
  Mercury sphygmomanometer with bladder and cuff

Equipment Preparation

- With mercury manometers, be sure the mercury column is at zero and falls freely when the pressure is released before beginning the blood pressure assessment.
- Check the parts of the sphygmomanometer.
    The valve should be clean and free to adjust in either direction.
    The pressure bulb should be free of leaks.
- Choose the appropriate size of cuff for the individual client. The width of the bladder within the cuff is ideally 40% of the circumference of the midpoint of the limb, or 20% wider than the diameter; a bladder 5 to 5½ inches (12 to 14 cm) is satisfactory for the average adult.

Client Preparation

- Be sure the room is warm and quiet. Have the client assume a sitting or lying position. (Optionally, take several readings with the client alternating sitting and lying to measure effects of postural changes.)
- Explain the procedure and have the client rest at least 5 minutes before measurement.
- At a client's first assessment, measure blood pressure in both arms; thereafter, take measurements in the arm with the higher pressure (a difference of 5 to 10 mm Hg is normal; a greater

difference may indicate a condition such as aortic stenosis or arterial occlusion).

The length of the bladder should be about twice the recommended width; the bladder should nearly encircle the arm.

History

- Assess for factors that normally influence blood pressure (Table 8).

Assessing Blood Pressure by Auscultation
Definition of Korotkoff Sounds

The Korotkoff sounds are auscultatory sounds heard over the artery as pressure in the cuff is gradually lowered from well above the systolic pressure and the collapsed artery reopens.

First sound—clear rhythmic tapping that gradually increases in intensity. Systolic pressure is the reading at the point the sound first appears.

Second sound—murmur or swishing as the vessel distends and blood creates vibrations in the vessel wall.

Third sound—movement of blood in the vessel sounds crisper and more intense, as the vessel remains open in systole but is obliterated in diastole.

Fourth sound—sound is muffled, as the cuff pressure falls below the blood pressure. (Often institutions use the fourth sound as diastolic pressure for children, and some use this point also for adults.)

Fifth sound—disappearance of sounds. Diastolic pressure is the reading at the point the sounds disappear.

Assessment Techniques—Auscultation

Procedure	Rationale
Assemble sphygmomanometer and stethoscope.	
Determine proper cuff size.	The proper cuff size is necessary to apply the correct amount of pressure over the artery.
Wash hands.	Remove microorganisms to avoid transmission to client.

Table 8   Factors that influence blood pressure

Factor	Effect
Age	Normal arterial pressure (systolic/diastolic)
	Newborn 50-52/25-30
	4 years 85/60
	6 years 95/62
	10 years 100/65
	12 years 108/67
	16 years 118/75
	Adult 120/80
Anxiety, fear, pain, and emotional stress	Increases blood pressure because of increased heart rate and increased peripheral vascular resistance.
Sex	After puberty, because of hormonal variations blood pressure in males increases; after menopause, blood pressure in women increases.
Medications	Blood pressure is lowered by antihypertensive and diuretic agents, certain antiarrhythmics, narcotic analgesics, and general anesthetics.
Diurnal variation	Blood pressure generally rises during the morning and afternoon and drops through the evening and night; individuals vary significantly.

Procedure	Rationale
Assist client to a comfortable sitting position, with arm slightly flexed, forearm supported at heart level, and palm turned up.	Arm above heart level produces false low reading. Position facilitates cuff application.

Procedure	Rationale
Expose upper arm fully.	Ensures proper cuff application.
Palpate brachial artery.	Cuff is to be positioned 1 inch (2.5 cm) above site of brachial artery pulsation (antecubital space).
Center the arrows marked on the cuff over the brachial artery.	Bladder should inflate directly over brachial artery to ensure that proper pressure is applied during inflation.
Be sure cuff is fully deflated. Wrap the cuff evenly and snugly around the upper arm.	Ensures that proper pressure will be applied over artery.
Be sure manometer is positioned vertically at eye level.	Prevents inaccurate reading of mercury level.
If unaware of client's normal systolic pressure, palpate radial artery and inflate cuff to a pressure 30 mm Hg above point at which radial pulsation disappears. Slowly deflate cuff and note when pulse reappears.	Identifies approximate systolic pressure and determines maximal inflation point for accurate reading. Prevents auscultatory gap.
Deflate cuff and wait 30 seconds.	Prevents venous congestion and false high readings.
Place stethoscope earpieces in the ears and be sure sounds are clear, not muffled.	Earpieces should follow angle of examiner's ear canal to facilitate hearing.
Relocate brachial artery and place diaphragm of stethoscope over it.	Stethoscope placement ensures optimum sound reception.
Close valve of pressure bulb clockwise until tight.	Prevents air leak during inflation.
Inflate cuff to pressure 30 mm Hg above client's normal systolic level.	Ensures accurate pressure measurement.

Procedure	Rationale
Slowly release valve, allowing mercury to fall at rate of 2 to 3 mm Hg per second.	Too rapid or too slow a decline in the mercury level may lead to inaccurate pressure readings.
Note point on manometer when first clear sound is heard.	The first Korotkoff sound indicates the systolic pressure.
Continue to deflate cuff gradually, noting the point when a muffled or dampened sound appears.	The fourth Korotkoff sound may be recorded in adults with hypertension, and the American Heart Association recommends the fourth Korotkoff sound as the indication of diastolic pressure in children.
Continue cuff deflation noting the point on the manometer when sound disappears.	The American Heart Association recommends recording the fifth Korotkoff sound as the diastolic pressure in adults.
Deflate cuff rapidly and remove from client's arm unless there is a need to repeat the measurement.	Continuous cuff inflation causes arterial occlusion, which results in numbness and tingling of the client's arm.
Wait 30 seconds before repeating procedure.	Prevents venous congestion and false high reading.
Fold cuff and store properly.	Proper maintenance of supplies ensures instrument accuracy.
Assist client to a preferred position and cover the upper arm.	Maintains client's comfort.
Compare blood pressure reading with previous baseline or normal values for client's age.	Evaluates for change in condition or presence of alterations.
Record in medical record or flow sheet.	Record vital signs immediately.

Common mistakes in auscultation method

Source of Error	Effect
Too wide a bladder or cuff	False low reading
Too narrow a bladder or cuff	False high reading
Cuff wrapped too loosely	False high reading
Deflating cuff too slowly	False high diastolic reading
Deflating cuff too quickly	False low systolic and false high diastolic reading
Stethoscope fits poorly or the examiner's hearing is impaired, causing sounds to be muffled	False low systolic and false high diastolic reading
Inaccurate inflation level	False low systolic reading
Multiple examiners using different Korotkoff sounds	Inaccurate interpretation of systolic and diastolic readings

Assessing Blood Pressure in Children

- Select cuff following same criteria as for adults; the bladder should completely or nearly encircle the extremity.
- Infants and children younger than 5 years of age should lie supine with arms supported at heart level; older children may sit.
- Keep the child relaxed and calm; wait at least 15 minutes after any activity or anxiety.
- Use same technique of auscultation as with adults.
- If auscultatory sounds are too faint to hear, use an ultrasonic stethoscope.

Assessing Blood Pressure by Palpation

The palpation method is used with clients whose arterial pulse is too weak to create Korotkoff's sounds, such as occurs with severe blood loss or weakened myocardial contractility.

- Apply blood pressure cuff in same manner as with auscultation method.
- Palpate the radial artery throughout the procedure instead of using a stethoscope.
- Raise the cuff pressure to 200 mm Hg or to 30 mm Hg above the client's usual systolic pressure.
- Allow the pressure to fall at about 2 mm Hg per second.

- The systolic pressure is the reading at which the radial pulse can again be palpated.
- The diastolic pressure, usually very difficult to palpate, feels like a thin snapping vibration.

Assessing Blood Pressure in Lower Extremities

It is necessary to measure blood pressure in the leg if accessibility to the arm is blocked by a dressing, cast, catheter, or other device or if the client has an abnormality that may cause a variation in blood pressure between the upper and lower extremities.

- The popliteal artery behind the knee is the auscultatory site.
- Position the client lying flat on the abdomen or, if necessary, sitting with knee flexed slightly for easier accessibility to the artery.
- Use a wide, long cuff; wrap the cuff so that the bladder is over the posterior aspect of the midthigh.
- Follow the same procedure as with brachial artery auscultation. NOTE: Systolic pressure in the legs is usually 10 to 40 mm Hg higher than in the brachial artery; diastolic pressure is usually about the same in both sites.

Client Teaching

- Before assessing clients' blood pressures, ask whether the clients know their normal blood pressures; if not, inform them of the measurements.
- Adult clients should have their blood pressure assessed at least once a year.
- Clients should be educated about hypertension risk factors:
    Obesity (>30% overweight)
    Smoking more than 10 cigarettes daily
    Heavy alcohol consumption
    High blood cholesterol levels (total cholesterol ≥240 mg/dL or LDL cholesterol ≥160 mg/dL)
    Continued exposure to stress
- Clients with hypertension should learn about blood pressure values, long-term, follow-up care and therapy, the usual lack of symptoms, therapy's ability to control and its inability to cure, and the importance of a consistently followed treatment plan to provide a relatively normal life-style (Joint National Committee on Detection, Evaluation, and Treatment of High Blood Pressure, 1984).

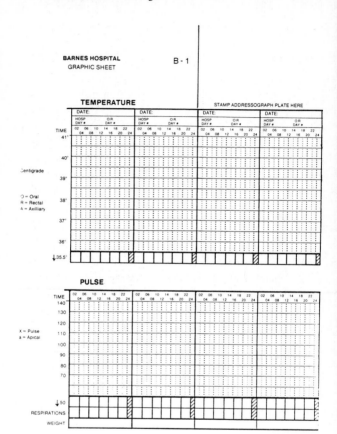

Fig. 9
Vital signs graphic sheet.
(Courtesy Barnes Hospital, St Louis, Mo.)

Guidelines for Recording and Reporting Vital Signs

- Institutional settings often have policies that prescribe ranges at which vital signs are to be reported to the physician.
- All vital sign measurements must be appropriately recorded and abnormalities must be appropriately reported.
- Special graphs, such as those shown in Fig. 9, allow recording of vital signs along with significant information regarding symptoms, interventions initiated, and notes on vital sign changes.
- Any significant change in a client's vital signs at any time should be reported to appropriate personnel.

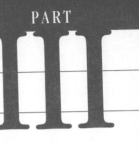

BODY
SYSTEM
ASSESSMENT

PART

III

Integument

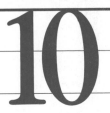

10

The integument provides external protection for the body, helps regulate body temperature, and is a sensory organ for pain, temperature, and touch. The integument may be assessed while the nurse assesses other body systems or at the beginning of the examination. Assessment includes skin, nails, hair, and scalp, using the skills of inspection and palpation.

Skin
Anatomy and Physiology

The main layers of the skin are the superficial epidermis and the thicker underlying dermis (Fig. 10). The epidermis consists of two layers: one containing dead cells and the other containing rapidly producing cells that replace cells lost during normal desquamation. The epidermis resurfaces wounds and restores a barrier to invading organisms. The dermis is elastic and durable and contains a complex network of nerve endings, sweat glands, sebaceous glands, hair follicles, and blood vessels. The skin insulates the body against extremes of cold and facilitates heat loss. When the body's temperature rises, the skin acts as a radiator promoting the radiation of heat that reaches the dermis by way of vasodilation and by providing a surface for the evaporation of sweat.

A third layer of subcutaneous tissue contains blood vessels, nerves, lymph, and loose connective tissue filled with fat cells. The fatty tissue serves as a heat insulator and provides support for upper skin layers.

Rationale

The skin is assessed for the following reasons:
1. Any break or disruption of the skin predisposes the person to infection.
2. The hydration of the skin and mucous membranes may reveal the body's regulation of body temperature.

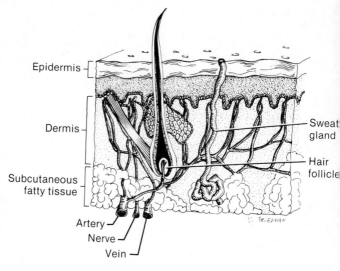

Fig. 10
Cross section of skin reveals three layers: epidermis, dermis, and subcutaneous fatty tissue.

3. Skin temperature changes can reflect alterations in blood flow.
4. Specific skin conditions or underlying diseases may be detected.
5. Condition of the skin reflects level of a person's hygiene.

Skin Assessment
Special equipment

The following equipment is used in assessing the skin:
Adequate lighting
Disposable gloves (for moist or draining lesions)

Client preparation

- For a total assessment of all skin surfaces the client must assume several positions.
- The area to be examined must be fully exposed.
- If an area is not clean, cleanse the skin before inspection.

History

- Ask the client about changes in skin color, the presence of lesions, and bruising.
- Ask whether the client works or spends excessive time outside.
- Ask about the frequency of bathing and the type of soap used.
- Ask whether there has been recent trauma to the skin.
- Ask whether the client has a history of allergies.
- Ask whether the client uses topical medications or home remedies (soaks or heating pads).
- Ask whether the client goes to tanning parlors, uses sun lamps, or lies in the sun frequently.

Assessment techniques

Assessment	Normal Findings
Inspect the skin for color and pigmentation (Table 9).	Normal pigmentation varies from light pink to ruddy pink in white skin; light to deep brown or olive in dark skin.
Note any patches or areas of skin with color variations.	With sun exposure some areas, such as the face and arms, have greater pigmentation.
Inspect lips, nail beds, and palms for cyanosis.	Dark-skinned clients have lighter-colored palms, soles, lips, and nail beds.
Inspect the sclera for jaundice.	Sclera is usually the color of white porcelain in white clients and light yellow in black clients.
Use fingertips to feel skin's moisture.	Skin is normally dry and warm.
Palpate skin temperature with the dorsum or the back of the hand.	
Stroke skin lightly with fingertips to determine texture.	Skin texture not normally consistent throughout body.

Continued on p. 87.

Table 9   Skin color variations

Color	Condition	Cause	Assessment Location
Bluing (cyanosis)	Increased amount of deoxygenated hemoglobin, associated with hypoxia	Heart or lung disease; cold environment	Nail beds; lips; mouth; skin (severe cases)
Pallor (decrease in color)	Reduced amount of oxyhemoglobin	Anemia	Face; conjunctiva; nail beds
	Reduced visibility of oxyhemoglobin as a result of decreased blood flow	Shock	Skin; nail beds; conjunctiva; lips
	Congenital or autoimmune condition causing lack of pigment	Vitiligo	Patchy areas on skin
Yellow-orange (jaundice)	Increased deposition of bilirubin in the tissues	Liver disease; destruction of red blood cells	Sclera; mucous membranes; skin
Red (erythema)	Increased visibility of oxyhemoglobin as a result of dilation or increased blood flow	Fever; direct trauma; blushing; alcohol intake	Face; area of trauma
Tan-brown	Increased amount of melanin	Suntan; pregnancy	Areas exposed to sun; face; areola; nipples

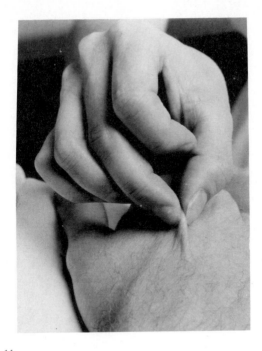

Fig. 11
Assessment for skin turgor
(From Potter PA and Perry AG: Fundamentals of nursing: process, concepts, and practice, ed 2, St Louis, 1989, The CV Mosby Co.)

Assessment	Normal Findings
Assess turgor by grasping a skin fold on the back of the hand or forearm and release. Note how easily the skin moves and snaps back into place (Fig. 11).	Normally the skin snaps back immediately to resting position.
Inspect any lesion for color, size, location, type, grouping, and distribution. Palpate gently using gloves if lesion is moist or draining (Table 10).	

Continued on p. 90.

Table 10 Skin lesions

Type	Size	Description	Example
Primary			
Macule	Less than ½ in (1 cm)	Flat; nonpalpable; change in skin color	Freckle; petechiae
Papule	Less than ¼ in (0.5 cm)	Palpable; circumscribed; solid elevation in skin	Elevated; nevus
Nodule	¼-1 in (0.5-2.5 cm)	Elevated solid mass; deeper and firmer than papule	Wart
Tumor	Larger than ½ -1 in (1-2.5 cm)	Solid mass, may extend deep through subcutaneous tissue	Epithelioma
Wheal	Varies	Elevated area of superficial localized edema; irregularly shaped	Hives; mosquito bite

Vesicle	Less than ¼ in (0.5 cm)	Circumscribed elevation of skin filled with serous fluid	Herpes simplex (chickenpox)
Pustule	Varies	Similar to vesicle; lesion filled with pus	Acne; *Staphylococcus* infection
Secondary Ulcer	Varies	Deep loss of skin surface; may extend to dermis; frequently bleeds and scars	Venous stasis ulcer
Atrophy	Varies	Thinning of skin with loss of normal skin furrow; skin appears shiny and translucent	Arterial insufficiency

Assessment	Normal Findings
Inspect any edematous areas for location, color, and shape. Skin may be stretched and shiny. Palpate any area of edema for mobility, consistency, and tenderness. To assess pitting edema, press the area firmly with thumb for 5 seconds and release; record depth of pitting in inches (centimeters). For example, 1+ edema equals depth of 1 cm and 2+ edema equals depth of 2 cm.	Normally skin is free of edema.

Deviations from Normal	Nurse Alert
Very dry skin may indicate dehydration or use of excessive soap. Perspiration indicates body's attempt to lose heat. Record color, odor, amount, and consistency of any fluid from lesions.	
Localized warmth around wound site may indicate inflammation or infection. Coldness of fingers may indicate reduced blood flow caused by temperature extremes, vascular disease, or vascular surgery.	Assess temperature with clients at risk for impaired circulation, that is, those with a tight cast or dressing.
Localized changes such as rash, inflammation, or swelling may result from an allergic reaction to cosmetics.	
Localized skin texture changes may result from trauma or lesions.	

Deviations from Normal	Nurse Alert
Skin turgor may be diminished by edema or dehydration. Dependent edema (typically in feet, ankles, and sacrum) may indicate poor venous return.	Puts client at risk for skin breakdown.
With irregular findings in texture or with lesions, ask client about changes. Changes in color or size of lesions may be precancerous signs. Localized areas of hardness beneath the skin may be a result of repeated intramuscular or subcutaneous injections, such as with a diabetic client or a client receiving vitamin B_{12} injections.	Instruct client on importance of rotating injection sites.

Nursing diagnosis

- Assessment data may reveal the following nursing diagnoses:
    Impaired skin integrity related to pressure on dependent areas or exposure to excretions.
    Potential impaired skin integrity related to immobilization.
    Altered health maintenance related to inability to perform hygiene.

Pediatric considerations

Skin rashes are common in infants because of food allergies. Developmental changes may cause skin changes such as facial acne in adolescents.

Gerontologic considerations

With increasing age, normal changes include graying and loss of scalp hair, skin wrinkling, decreased skin turgor, and decreased hair on extremities and axillary and pubic areas. Skin may be drier because of diminished sebaceous and sweat gland activity. Facial hair may become coarser and more apparent in women.

A common skin lesion that develops with aging is seborrheic

or senile keratosis. This is a benign growth appearing on the trunk, face, and scalp as single or multiple lesions. It is a superficial, circumscribed, raised area that thickens and darkens over time.

Actinic keratosis, common in men past middle age, is a lesion that can become cancerous. It appears in areas exposed to the sun, such as bald heads, hands, and faces. The lesion is a localized thickening of the skin that begins as a reddish, scaly, superficial area.

Client teaching

- Instruct client how to prevent skin cancer by avoiding overexposure to the sun: wear wide-brimmed hats and long sleeves, use sunscreens before going in the sun and after swimming or perspiring, avoid tanning at midday (11 AM to 2 PM).
- Teach the client to conduct a monthly self-examination of the skin, noting any moles, blemishes, or birthmarks.
- Tell the client to report any changes in the size, shape, or color of lesions. If a sore does not heal, report it to a physician.
- The elderly tend to have delayed wound healing. Instruct the client to report to a physician any lesions that bleed or fail to heal.
- Teach the client to avoid applying drying agents such as rubbing alcohol or soap to the skin.
- Tell the client to apply lotion and moisturizer to the skin regularly to reduce itching and drying.
- Inform the client that baths need not be taken daily.
- Instruct adolescents on proper skin cleansing and the importance of a balanced diet and adequate rest.

Nails
Anatomy and Physiology

The most visible portion of the nails is the nail plate, the transparent layer of epithelial cells covering the nail bed. The vascularity of the nail bed creates the nail's underlying color. The semilunar, whitish area at the base of the nail bed from which the nail plate develops is called the lunula.

Rationale

The condition of the nails can reflect a person's general health.

Nail Assessment
Special equipment

The following equipment is used in assessing the nails:
Adequate lighting

Client preparation

- Performed during skin assessment.

History

- Ask whether the client has experienced recent trauma to the nails.
- Determine the client's nail care practices.
- Ask whether the client has noticed changes in nail appearance or growth.
- Ask the parents whether a pediatric client nail-bites.

Assessment techniques

Assessment	Normal Findings
Inspect the nail bed color, the thickness and shape of the nail, the angle between the nail and the nail bed, and the condition of tissue around the nail.	Nails normally are transparent, smooth, and convex, with pink nail beds and translucent white tips. In blacks, brown or black pigmentation is normal between fingernail and nail base. Normal angle of the nail bed is 160 degrees.
Palpate the nail base.	Nail bed is normally firm.
Assess adequacy of circulation and capillary refill by palpation: apply gentle, firm pressure with thumb to nail bed. Release pressure quickly.	White color of nail bed under pressure should instantly return to pink.

Deviations from Normal

Nail growth may be impaired by direct injury or generalized disease.
Blue or purple coloration of nail bed may indicate cyanosis.
White pallor of nail bed results from anemia.
Thin nails may indicate nutritional deficiency.

Table 11   Abnormalities of the nail bed

Type	Description
Clubbing	Change occurs in the angle between nail and nail base because of long-term reduction in oxygenation to tissues. The nail bed softens, with the nail flattening. Eventually the angle is greater than 180 degrees. The fingertips often become enlarged.
Beau's lines	Transverse depressions in the nails, indicating that nail growth was temporarily disturbed. Grows out over several months.
Koilonychia (spoon nail)	Concave curves.
Splinter hemorrhages	Red or brown linear streaks in the nail bed.
Paronychia	Inflammation of skin at base of nail.

Deviations from Normal

Changes in shape or curvature of nails indicate systemic disease.
Failure of pinkness to return to nail bed after pressure is applied and released indicates circulatory insufficiency.
Ragged, short nails may indicate nail-biting.
See Table 11 for abnormalities of the nail bed.

Gerontologic considerations

With age, the nails of the fingers and toes develop longitudinal striations. The rate of nail growth slows.

Client teaching

- Nail polish and nail polish remover cause drying and brittleness of nails and cuticles.
- Instruct client to cut nails only after soaking them about 10 minutes in warm water.
- Caution client against use of over-the-counter preparations to treat corns, calluses, or ingrown toenails.

- Tell client to cut nails straight across and even with tops of fingers and toes.
- Nails should be shaped with a file or emery board.

Hair and Scalp
Anatomy and Physiology

Two types of hair cover the body, terminal hair (long, coarse, thick hair easily visible on the scalp, axilla, and pubic areas) and vellus hair (small, soft, tiny hairs covering the whole body except for palms and soles).

Hair and Scalp Assessment
Special equipment

The following equipment is used in assessing the hair and scalp:
   Adequate lighting
   Disposable gloves (if lice are suspected)

Client preparation

- Assessment occurs during all portions of the examination.
- Explain the need to separate parts of hair to detect obvious problems.

History

- Ask whether the client is wearing a wig or hairpiece and request that it be removed.
- Determine whether the client has noted a change in hair growth or a loss of hair.
- Identify the type of shampoo, other hair care products, or curling irons used.
- Determine whether the client has recently received chemotherapy (if hair loss is noted).

Assessment techniques

Assessment	Normal Findings
Inspect the distribution, thickness, texture, and lubrication of body hair.	Hair is normally distributed evenly, is neither excessively dry nor oily, and is pliant.

Assessment	Normal Findings
	Asian and black Americans have less hair than whites, and Native Americans have little or no hair on their bodies.
Separate sections of scalp hair to observe characteristics.	Normal terminal hair is black, brown, red, yellow, or variations of these shades. The hair is coarse or fine.
	The hair of black clients is usually thicker, curlier, and drier than the hair of white clients.
Inspect the scalp for lesions, which easily go unnoticed in thick hair; separate hair at various locations for thorough examination.	Scalp is smooth and inelastic, with even coloration.
Inspect hair follicles on the scalp and pubic areas for lice or other parasites. Lice attach their eggs to hair. Avoid close contact of your uniform to prevent transmission of lice.	
Head and body lice are tiny and have grayish white bodies. Crab lice have red legs. Lice eggs look like oval particles of dandruff.	
Inspect follicles for bites or pustular eruptions.	

Deviations from Normal	Nurse Alert
Unusual distribution or growth of hair may indicate a hormone disorder.	Changes in hair growth or distribution can damage the client's body image and emotional well-being.
Females with hirsutism have hair on upper lip, chin, and cheeks and coarser vellus hair on the body.	

Deviations from Normal	Nurse Alert

Hair loss may result from scalp disease, disturbed body functions such as febrile illness, or administration of general anesthesia.

Excessively oily hair may result from androgen hormone stimulation.

Dry, coarse, or discolored hair may result from poor nutrition, and dry brittle hair may be caused by excessive use of shampoo or other chemical agents.

Reduced hair on extremities, particularly the legs, may result from arterial insufficiency.

Nursing diagnoses

▪ Assessment data may reveal the following nursing diagnoses:
    Body image disturbance related to hair loss.
    Potential for infection related to head lice.

Pediatric considerations

Localized loss of hair such as on the back of the head may indicate that the infant lies too frequently in one position and may have unmet stimulation needs.

During adolescence a change in the amount and distribution of hair growth occurs.

Gerontologic considerations

In the elderly, the hair becomes dull, gray, white, or yellow. It also thins over the scalp, axilla, and pubic areas. Elderly men lose facial hair, whereas elderly women may have hair growth on the chin and upper lip. With aging there is a reduction in hair covering the lower extremities.

Client teaching

▪ Clients may require instruction about basic hygiene measures, including shampooing and combing the hair.

- Instruct clients who have lice about the frequency of using Kwell shampoo or soap and the risks for transmitting infection.
- Instruct the client who has lice to notify sexual partners about the risk of transmitting lice during sexual contact.
- If scalp moles are found, instruct the client how to comb or brush hair to avoid bleeding.

Head

Before assessing particular structures and functions of the eyes, ears, nose and sinuses, mouth and pharynx, and neck, inspect the general appearance of the head.

Client Preparation

- Client assumes a sitting position.

History

- Determine whether the client has experienced recent trauma to the head.
- Ask whether the client has noticed neurologic symptoms such as headaches, dizziness, loss of consciousness, seizures, or blurred vision.
- Determine length of time the client has experienced neurologic symptoms.

Assessment Techniques

Assessment	Normal Findings
Inspect the head for size, shape, and contour.	The skull is generally round with prominence in the frontal area anteriorly and occipital area posteriorly.
Palpate the skull for nodules or masses by gently rotating fingertips down the midline of the scalp and then along the sides of the head.	Scalp overlying the skull is normally smooth and elastic.
With neonate, palpate anterior and posterior fontanels for size, shape, and texture.	Fontanels are normally flat, smooth, and well demarcated.

Deviations from Normal

Local skull deformities may result from trauma.

Large head in adults may result from excessive growth hormone (acromegaly).

Avoid applying pressure directly over fontanels because of potential for intracranial damage.

Pediatric Considerations

The posterior fontanel normally closes by the second month, and the anterior fontanel closes at 12 to 18 months of age. In infants, a large head may result from congenital anomalies or cerebrospinal fluid in the ventricles (hydrocephalus).

Client Teaching

Assure parents that open fontanels are normal and caution them to protect the neonate's skull from pressure and potential trauma.

Eyes

12

Anatomy and Physiology

The organs of sight are contained in a bony orbit at the front of the skull, embedded in orbital fat, and innervated by one of a pair of optic nerves from the brain's occipital lobes. Light enters the eye through the transparent cornea (Fig. 12). The lens changes shape to focus light on a layer of rods and cones constituting the retina. Impulses created by the retina's specialized nerve cells transmit a visual image along the optic nerve to the brain.

Rationale

Examination of the eye involves the assessment of four areas: visual acuity, visual fields, extraocular movements, and external structures. It also includes an ophthalmoscopic examination. The nurse determines the presence of visual symptoms that may indicate the presence of specific eye disorders. Any visual alterations can significantly affect a client's ability to remain independent in performing self-care activities.

Eye Assessment
Special Equipment

Newspaper or magazine
Index card
Snellen eye chart
Cotton-tipped applicator
Penlight
Ophthalmoscope
Small ruler

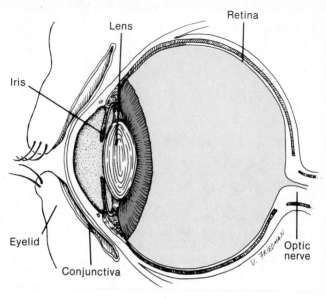

Fig. 12
Cross section of eye.

Client Preparation

- Throughout the examination the client is asked to sit or stand.
- The room may be darkened during the opthalmoscopic examination.

History

- Determine whether the client has history of eye disease, diabetes, or hypertension.
- Ask the client about presence of eye pain, photophobia (sensitivity to light), burning, itching, excess tearing or crusting, diplopia (double vision), blurred vision, floaters (small black spots that seem to cross the field of vision), flashing lights, or halos around lights.
- Assess client's occupational history for activities requiring close, intricate work or activities, such as welding, that create risk for eye injury.
- Ask the client whether glasses or contacts are normally worn.
- Determine date of the client's last eye examination.

Assessment Techniques
Visual acuity

Assessment of visual acuity can progress in stages, depending on the response in each stage and the reason for the assessment.

Stage I

Make cursory assessment by asking the client to read newspaper or magazine print. Be sure light is adequate. A client who wears glasses should wear them during this stage of assessment.

Be sure the client knows English and is literate. Asking the client to read aloud can help determine literacy. If the client has difficulty, proceed to Stage II.

Stage II

Test each eye by having the client read with index card covering one eye at a time. Do not use hand to cover eye. Ask clients with severe impairments to count upraised fingers or distinguish light. For more accurate assessment, proceed to Stage III.

Stage III

For accurate assessment, use Snellen eye chart. Have the client wear glasses unless they are only for reading. Have the client stand 20 feet from the eye chart. Ask the client to read the smallest possible line of print—once with both eyes open and once with each eye covered. Ability to read more than half the letters/numbers in a line correctly is considered a success for that line. With clients who are unable to read, use an "E" chart and indicate the direction the E's arms point. With young children, use a chart with images of familiar objects. Record visual acuity score for each eye as two numbers:

Numerator (20) = Feet from chart
Denominator = Standardized number for that line on the chart (example: 20/80). Distance from which the normal eye can read)

Normal Findings

Normal visual acuity is 20/20 for each eye.

Deviations from Normal	Nurse Alert
Visual acuity of 20/200 is considered legal blindness.	Clients with impaired visual acuity may require assistance in performing the activities of daily living. The client's ability to read educational materials may also be impaired.

Visual fields

Assessment	Normal Findings
Have the client stand 2 feet (60 cm) away, facing you.	
Make sure your eyes are at the client's eye level.	
Ask the client to cover one eye with index card and look at your eye directly opposite.	
Close or cover your eye opposite the client's closed eye.	
Hold your finger at arm's length to one side, midway between you and the client.	
Be sure finger is outside the field of vision, then slowly bring it back.	
Ask clients to say when they begin to see your finger.	Both you and the client should see your finger entering the field of vision at about the same point.
Bring your finger slowly closer, always keeping it midway between you and the client.	
Repeat procedure on the other side, then above, then below, always comparing the point at which you see the finger coming into your field of vision and the point at which the client sees it.	
Repeat procedure in all four directions with other eye.	

Deviations from Normal	Nurse Alert
If the client sees your finger significantly later than you do, the client may have altered visual fields.	Refer any client with visual field alterations to a physician or ophthalmologist for a detailed eye examination.
Visual field alterations (the blacking out of a portion of the field) are commonly caused by optic nerve damage or retinal disorders.	

Extraocular movements

The movement of each eye depends on six small muscles and the innervation of cranial nerves.

Assessment	Normal Findings
Have the client stand 2 feet away, facing you.	
Ask the client to follow the movement of your finger with both eyes.	
Ask the client not to turn or move his head.	
Keeping your finger about 6 to 12 inches from the client's face, move the finger smoothly and slowly through the eight cardinal gazes (Fig. 13): Up and down Right and left Diagonally up and down to left Diagonally up and down to right	
Keep the finger within the normal field of vision.	
Observe for parallel eye movement, the position of the upper eyelid in relation to the iris, and the presence of any abnormal movements.	The eyes should move smoothly and parallel in the direction of gaze. The upper eyelid covers the iris only slightly in all directions.

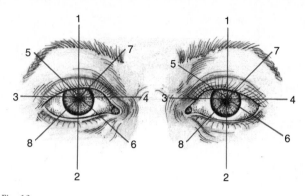

Fig. 13
The eight directions of gaze.
(From Potter PA and Perry AG: Fundamentals of nursing: process, concepts, and practice, ed 2, St Louis, 1989, The CV Mosby Co.)

Deviations from Normal	Nurse Alert
The upper eyelid covers much of the iris.	Altered eye movements can reflect injury or disease of eye muscles, supporting structures, or cranial nerves.
Presence of abnormal eye movements such as nystagmus (rhythmic oscillation of the eyes), which is often elicited by gaze to far left or right.	
Lacrimal apparatus:	*Lacrimal apparatus:*
For the remainder of the examination, the client's contact lenses should be removed.	
Inspect lacrimal gland area in upper outer wall of anterior part of orbit for edema or redness (Fig. 14).	Tears flow from the gland across the eye's surface to the lacrimal duct.
Palpate gland area gently to detect any tenderness.	The lacrimal gland area is nontender. The gland cannot normally be palpated.
Inspect lacrimal duct at the nasal corner (inner canthus) for edema or excess tearing.	

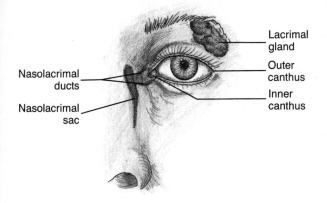

Fig. 14
Lacrimal apparatus.
(From Potter PA and Perry AG: Fundamentals of nursing: process, concepts, and practice ed 2, St Louis, 1989, The CV Mosby Co.)

Assessment	Normal Findings

Conjunctiva and sclera:
Gently retract eyelids to inspect conjunctiva as follows:
Avoid applying pressure directly on eyeball.
Gently depress lower lid with thumb against bony orbit and ask the client to look upward (Fig. 15).

Inspect conjunctiva's color and assess for edema or lesions.
Take special care in retracting upper lid (do not perform the first time without qualified assistance).

Ask the client to look down, relax eyes, and avoid sudden movements.
Gently grasp upper lid, pulling lashes down and forward.

Conjunctiva are transparent with light pink color.
The sclera has color of white porcelain in white clients and light yellow in black clients.

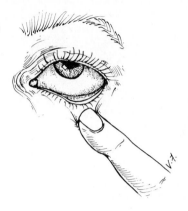

Fig. 15

Technique for retracing lower eyelid.

(From Potter PA and Perry AG: Fundamentals of nursing: process, concepts, and practice, ed 2, St Louis, 1989, The CV Mosby Co.)

Assessment	Normal Findings
Place tip of cotton-tipped applicator ½ inch (1 cm) above lid margin.	
Push down on upper eyelid to turn it inside out; keep lid inverted by careful grasp of upper lashes.	
Inspect conjunctiva for edema, lesions, or presence of foreign bodies.	
After inspection, return lid to normal position by gently pulling lashes forward and asking client to look up.	
Pupils and iris:	*Pupils and iris:*
Inspect pupil for size, shape, equality, and reaction to light.	Pupils are normally round and equal in size.
Inspect iris for margin defects.	

Assessment	Normal Findings
Test light reflex in dimly lit room: Bring penlight from side of client's face and direct light onto pupil as the client looks straight ahead. Observe illuminated pupil.	The illuminated pupil normally constricts briskly.
Continue to have client look straight ahead. Bring penlight from side of client's face and direct light on pupil (repeat for opposite side).	Pupil opposite the one illuminated constricts simultaneously.
Test accommodation reflex: Ask client to gaze at an object held 3 to 4 feet away and move object toward the client's nose.	Pupils converge and accommodate by constricting when looking at close objects. Pupil responses are equal.
Cornea: Standing at client's side inspect the cornea for clarity and texture. (Use oblique lighting.)	Cornea is normally shiny, transparent, and smooth.

Deviations from Normal

Position and alignment:

Bulging eyes (exophthalmos) usually indicates a thyroid disorder.

Strabismus (eyes crossed or gazing in different directions) is caused by neuromuscular injury or inherited anomalies.

Abnormal protrusion of one eye indicates possible tumor or inflammation of the eye's orbit.

Eyebrows:

Asymmetry.

Hair loss around eyebrows may be caused by hormonal deficiency.

Inability to move the eyebrows indicates a facial nerve paralysis.

Eyelids:

Abnormal drooping of the lid over the pupil (ptosis) can be caused by edema or third cranial nerve damage.

Deviations from Normal

Defects in lid margin position include ectropion (turning out of lid margin) and entropion (turning in of lid margin), which may cause irritation of conjunctiva.

Redness of lids indicates inflammation or infection.

Edema of eyelids, caused by heart or kidney failure or allergies, may impair ability of eyelids to close.

Inspect any lesions for characteristics, discomfort, or drainage.

Failure of eyelids to close completely is common in unconscious clients or those with facial nerve paralysis.

Lacrimal apparatus:

Swollen gland area, edema, or redness may indicate tumor, infection, or abscess.

Obstructed lacrimal duct may result in edema and excess tearing.

Conjunctiva and sclera:

Pale conjunctiva results from anemia.

Fiery red conjunctiva results from inflammation (conjunctivitis).

Pupils and iris:

Dilated or constricted pupils may result from neurologic disorders or medications.

Delayed or absent light or accommodation reflex may indicate changes in intracranial pressure, nerve lesions, ophthalmic medications, or direct trauma to eye.

Nurse Alert

Do not attempt to remove a foreign body that appears embedded in the conjunctiva but notify a physician immediately.

Clients suffering visual symptoms may be fearful of the potential loss of vision. Nurses should thus provide a thorough explanation of all examination procedures.

Nursing Diagnosis

Assessment data may reveal the following nursing diagnoses:
- Potential for injury related to reduced visual acuity and peripheral vision
- Sensory/perceptual alteration (visual) related to reduced visual acuity and visual changes of aging.
- Knowledge deficit regarding preventive eye care related to inexperience.

Pediatric Considerations

Abnormalities in placement or position of the eyes may indicate congenital alterations. Lacrimal apparatus is not present in infants until 3 months of age.

Gerontologic Considerations

With aging, the lacrimal glands decrease their production of tears causing the eyes to appear dry and lusterless. A common change is the presence of arcus senilis, a white ring that appears around the iris. Other changes include scleral discolorations, decrease in pupil size, decrease in peripheral vision, increase in the rate of dark adaptation, and clouding of the lens (cataract). The pupil may have an irregular shape in elderly clients.

Client Teaching

- School-age children require visual screening by age 3 or 4 years and every 2 years thereafter.
- Inform adult clients that persons younger than 40 years of age should have complete eye examinations every 3 to 5 years (or more often if family history reveals risks).
- Instruct clients older than 40 years of age to have eye examinations every 2 years to screen for glaucoma. Screening should also be done for presbyopia.
- Persons older than 65 years of age should have yearly eye examinations.
- Describe typical warning signs of eye disease.
- Clients with burning or itching of the eyes should avoid rubbing them to prevent transmitting infection from one eye to the other.
- Instruct clients on proper administration of eye drops and ointments. Instruct clients never to share medications with another person. Cleanse the eye by wiping from the inner to the outer canthus.
- Instruct elderly clients to take the following precautions because of normal visual changes: avoid driving at night, increase nonglare lighting in the home to reduce risk of falls, and look to sides before crossing streets.

Ophthalmoscopic Examination

The ophthalmoscope is used to inspect the fundus of the eye, including the retina, choroid, optic nerve disc, macula, fovea centralis, and retinal vessels.

Rationale

Ophthalmoscopic examination is particularly important for clients with diabetes, hypertension, or intracranial pathologic conditions.

Client Preparation

- Have client remove glasses. (Examiner should remove glasses too.)
- Conduct examination in a darkened room.
- Be sure you can handle the ophthalmoscope correctly and can recognize the normal appearance of the fundus.
- Position the dial so that the round white light is used.
- Stand facing the client with your eyes at the client's eye level.
- Ask the client to gaze straight ahead at an object slightly upward.
- Use right hand and eye to inspect the client's right eye and left hand and eye to inspect the client's left eye.

Assessment Techniques

Assessment	Normal Findings
Begin by standing slightly to the client's right. Keep both eyes open while looking through keyhole viewer. Set diopter at 0. Hold the ophthalmoscope firmly against your head and look through the ophthalmoscope about 10 inches (25 cm) from the client's eye as the light shines toward the pupil.	
Move in slowly, keeping the light on the red reflex (bright orange glow in the pupil).	Red reflex normally uniform and brilliant.
Rotate the lens disc to focus on the eye's internal structures.	3 to 5 cm from the eye, retinal structures become visible.

Assessment	Normal Findings
Assess the size, color, and clarity of the disc; the integrity of vessels; any retinal lesions; and the appearance of the macula and fovea.	Clear, yellow optic nerve disc. Reddish pink retina. Light red arteries and dark red veins. Vein size about 1½ times artery size. Avascular macula.

Deviations from Normal	Nurse Alert
With any deviations from normal findings, such as narrowing of vessels and changes in pigment of macula or optic nerve disc, refer client to an ophthalmologist.	Because the bright light of the ophthalmoscope is irritating and can cause tearing, do not illuminate the fundus too long. Ask clients to tell you if they become uncomfortable.

Nursing diagnosis

See previous diagnosis following eye assessment.

Client teaching

See previous teaching recommendations following eye assessment.

Pediatric considerations

Because a child may be fearful of the equipment and the dark, the nurse should show the ophthalmoscope to the child and explain the procedure before beginning.

Gerontologic considerations

With aging the retinal arterioles become pale and narrowed.

Ears

13

Assessment of the ears includes inspection of the auricle, otoscopic examination of the outer and middle ear, and hearing acuity tests, described separately below.

Anatomy and Physiology

The organ of hearing consists of the external, middle, and inner ear (Fig. 16). Sound waves transmitted by way of the external auditory canal cause the sensitive tympanic membrane to vibrate and conduct sound waves through the bony ossicles to the sensory organs of the inner ear. The semicircular canals, vestibule, and cochlea within the inner ear are the sensory structures for hearing and balance. Sound waves travel from the inner ear along the eighth cranial nerve to the brain.

Rationale

The nurse assesses the ears to determine the integrity of ear structures and the condition of hearing. Ear disorders may result from mechanical dysfunction or blockage, trauma caused by foreign bodies or high noise levels, damage to the auditory nerve, or acute illness such as viral infections, all of which should be considered during the ear assessment.

Ear Assessment
Special Equipment

Otoscope
Ear speculum
Tuning fork (256, 512, or 1024 Hz)

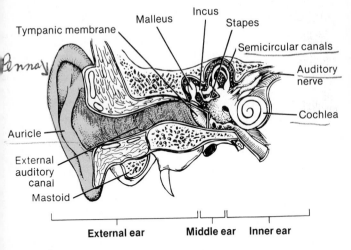

Fig. 16
Ear structures. External ear consists of auricle and external
auditory canal. Middle ear structures include tympanic
membrane and bony ossicles (malleus, incus, and stapes).
Inner ear includes semicircular canal, cochlea, and auditory
nerves.

Client Preparation

- Have the client sit during the examination.
- During the otoscopic examination choose the proper size ear
  speculum (largest that fits comfortably in ear).

History

- Has the client experienced ear pain, itching, discharge, tinnitus
  (ringing in ears), vertigo, or change in hearing?
- Assess risks for hearing problems (varies by age-group), including hypoxia at birth, meningitis, birth weight less than
  1500 grams, family history of hearing loss, congenital anomalies of the skull or face, nonbacterial intrauterine infections (rubella and herpes), and constant exposure to noise.
- Has client had ear surgery or trauma?
- Determine the client's exposure to loud noises at work and the
  availability of protective devices.
- Note behaviors indicative of hearing loss, including failure to

respond when spoken to, repetition of the question, "What did you say?", leaning forward to hear, and inattentiveness in children.

- Ask whether the client takes large doses of aspirin or antibiotics.
- Determine whether the client uses a hearing aid.

Assessment Techniques
Inspection of auricle

Assessment	Normal Findings
Inspect the auricle's placement, color, size, and symmetry and compare with normal findings.	The auricles are of equal size and level with each other with the upper point of attachment at the level of the lateral canthus of the eye. The color should be the same as the face.
Gently palpate the auricle for texture, lumps, or skin lesions.	Auricle is normally smooth without lesions.
Palpate the mastoid process for tenderness and temperature	Painless and warm during palpation.
If the ear seems inflamed or the client has pain, pull on the auricle and press on the tragus to detect increased pain.	Pulling on the auricle normally is painless. If pulling the auricle fails to aggravate existing pain, the client may have a middle ear infection.
Inspect the size of the external auditory meatus and note any discharge.	The meatus should not be swollen or occluded. Yellow waxy cerumen is common.

Deviations from Normal

Low-set ears may indicate a congenital abnormality.

Redness of the auricle may indicate inflammation or fever. A pale auricle can indicate frostbite.

Deviations from Normal

Pain in the external ear on palpation may indicate an external ear infection.

Yellowish or greenish discharge indicates infection.

Otoscopic examination

Assessment	Normal Findings
Check canal opening for foreign bodies before inserting speculum.	The ear canal is free of lesions, discharge, and inflammation.
Ask client to avoid any head movement to avoid damage to canal and tympanic membrane.	
Ask client to tip head toward opposite shoulder.	
Straighten the ear canal in adults and older children by pulling the auricle upward and backward (in infants, backward and downward).	
Insert the speculum into the canal slightly down and forward. Do not abrade the canal lining.	
Brace the otoscope against the client's head.	
Avoid any sudden movement.	
Inspect canal for color, lesions, foreign bodies, and discharge.	Cerumen may be yellow, dark red, black, or brown with a flaky, waxy, soft or hard consistency.
	Cerumen is odorless.
	Canal walls are pink and nontender.

Assessment	Normal Findings
Inspect ear drum (tympanic membrane) by moving the otoscope to see the entire drum and its periphery.	The ear drum is translucent, shiny, and pearly gray. The tympanic membrane is free of tears or breaks (Fig. 17). The bony prominence of the malleus can be seen in the center of the ear drum at the umbo. The light from the otoscope appears as a cone. The membrane may move during swallowing.

Deviations from Normal	Nurse Alert
A reddened ear canal is a sign of inflammation. Foul-smelling drainage indicates infection. Blood may be behind the eardrum if it appears dull with a bluish color. A pink or red membrane indicates inflammation. Perforations or scarring is abnormal.	If a foreign body is present in the ear canal, be careful not to impact the body farther into the ear canal with the otoscope. With impacted foreign bodies, a physician or other specialist should perform the removal.

Hearing acuity

Assessment	Normal Findings
Simple screening test:	
Test one ear at a time, asking client to occlude other ear with a finger. Stand about 1 foot (30 cm) from client.	
Exhale fully first and whisper random numbers to the client, covering your mouth with your hand to prevent the client from lipreading.	Clients normally hear numbers clearly when whispered.

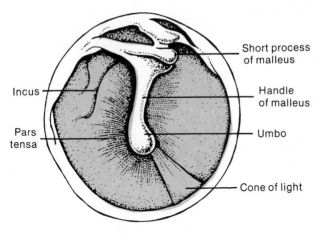

Fig. 17
Normal tympanic membrane.

Assessment	Normal Findings
Ask client to repeat the numbers.	
If necessary, gradually increase the loudness of the whisper.	
Test other ear and note any difference.	
A ticking watch may be held over the ear instead of whispering.	Clients normally hear a watch tick from 1 to 2 inches away.
	If a client has difficulty hearing, test further with tuning fork test.
Weber test for conduction deafness: (Fig. 18)	*Weber test for conduction deafness:*
Hold tuning fork by its base and strike it against palm or knuckle of opposite hand.	Client hears tuning fork equally in both ears or at midline of head.
Place base of vibrating fork on center of top of client's head.	

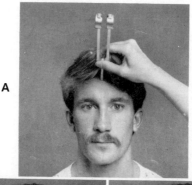

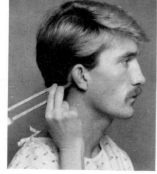 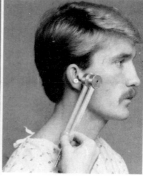

Fig. 18
Using a tuning fork to assess auditory function. **A,** Weber
test. **B** and **C,** Rinne's test.
(From Potter PA and Perry AG: Fundamentals of nursing: concepts, process, and
practice, ed 2, St Louis, 1989, The CV Mosby Co.)

Assessment	Normal Findings
Ask clients where they best hear the sound.	
Rinne test to compare air and bone conduction: (Fig. 18)	*Rinne test to compare air and bone conduction:*
Hold tuning fork by its base and strike it against palm or knuckle of opposite hand.	Air conduction hearing is normally twice as long as bone conduction hearing (positive Rinne).

Assessment	Normal Findings
Touch the base of the vibrating fork to the client's mastoid process and ask the client to tell you when the sound is no longer heard.	
Then place vibrating fork close to external meatus of one ear.	
Ask whether the client can hear the sound.	
Repeat with other ear.	

Deviations from Normal	Nurse Alert

Deviations from Normal	Nurse Alert
Weber test: Clients with air conduction deafness hear the tuning fork better in the affected ear because bone transmits sound directly to ear. *Rinne test:* Clients with air conduction deafness hear tuning fork better through bone conduction (negative Rinne).	Clients with impaired hearing should be referred to their physician for further evaluation. To minimize communication problems, stand to the side of the client's better ear, speak in a clear, normal tone of voice, and face the client so that your lips and face can be seen.

Nursing Diagnosis

Assessment data may reveal the following diagnoses:
- Sensory/perceptual alterations (auditory) related to impacted cerumen, inflamed ear canal, or trauma.
- Knowledge deficit regarding ear care related to information misinterpreted.
- Potential for injury related to hearing impairment.

Pediatric Considerations

Before otoscopic examination, be sure the child has not placed a foreign body in the ear. Young children may need to be restrained or held by the parent with head immobile. Infants should lie supine with the head turned to one side and arms held securely at the sides. Parents should be informed to teach children not to put foreign objects in their ears.

Gerontologic Considerations

Because of changes in sebaceous glands, itching of the ear canal may be a problem for some older adults. Excessive scratching or rubbing, which may lead to inflammation, should be avoided.

Elderly people often have a reduced ability to hear high-frequency sounds and consonant sounds such as S, Z, T, and G.

Deterioration of the cochlea and thickening of the tympanic membrane cause a gradual loss in hearing.

Client Teaching

- Instruct the client about the proper way to clean the outer ear with a damp cloth and about avoiding use of cotton-tipped applicators and sharp objects such as hair pins.
- Tell the client to avoid inserting pointed objects into the ear canal.
- Children should have routine ear screenings. Clients older than 65 years of age should have their hearing checked regularly.
- Instruct family members of clients with hearing losses to speak in normal low tones and not to shout.
- Instruct clients to get safety measures such as wake-up and burglar alarms, doorbells, smoke detectors, or telephones connected to a flashing light.
- Explore use of a hearing aid with the client.

Nose and Sinuses

14

Anatomy and Physiology

The nose consists of an internal and an external portion. The external portion is considerably smaller than the internal portion, which lies over the roof of the mouth. The interior of the nose is hollow and is separated by a partition, the septum, into a right and a left cavity. Each nasal cavity is divided into three passageways (superior, middle, and inferior meatus) by the projection of the turbinates (conchae) from the lateral walls of the internal portion of the nose. The technical name for the external openings into the nasal cavities (nostrils) is *anterior nares.*

The posterior nares (choanae) are openings from an area of the internal nasal cavity above the superior meatus, called the sphenoethmoidal recess, into the nasopharynx.

The nose serves as a passageway for air going to and from the lungs, filtering it of impurities and warming, moistening, and chemically examining it for substances that might prove irritating to the mucous lining of the respiratory tract. It serves as the organ of smell, since olfactory receptors are located in the nasal mucosa, and it aids in phonation.

Rationale

The nurse inspects the nose to determine symmetry of structures and presence of inflammation or infection.

Nose and Sinus Assessment
Special Equipment

Nasal speculum
Penlight

Client Preparation

- The client may sit.

History

- Ask whether the client experienced recent trauma or surgery to the nose.
- Ask whether the client has allergies, nasal discharge, epistaxis, frequent infections, headaches, or postnasal drip.
- Ask whether the client uses a nasal spray or drops.
- Ask whether the client snores or has difficulty breathing.

Assessment Techniques
Nose

Assessment	Normal Findings
Inspect external nose for shape and skin appearance. Note any deformity or inflammation.	Nose is smooth and symmetric with same color as face.
Gently palpate for tenderness and underlying deviation.	No pain on palpation.
Use penlight to examine each naris grossly.	
To insert a speculum have the client tip the head backward. Hold speculum in hand and brace it with your index finger against the client's nose. Insert speculum about 1 cm to dilate naris. Use other hand to hold penlight.	
With penlight and nasal speculum, inspect mucosa for color, lesions, discharge, swelling, or evidence of recent bleeding.	Normal mucosa is pink and moist. Discharge resulting from sinus irritation is clear and watery.
For client with a nasogastric tube, inspect for local excoriation, redness, and skin sloughing.	

Assessment	Normal Findings
Inspect septum and turbinates for deviation, lesions, and superficial blood vessels.	Turbinates are the same color as the mucosa, are moist, and are without lesions. The septum is symmetric.
Palpate sinuses with gentle upward pressure in frontal and maxillary areas.	Sinuses are normally non-tender.

Deviations from Normal	Nurse Alert
Edema and discoloration may result from recent trauma. Yellow or greenish discharge may indicate sinus infection. Pale mucosa with clear discharge indicates allergy. Inflamed, swollen, tender sinuses indicate infection or allergy. Polyps, lesions, or bleeding of turbinates is abnormal.	A deviated septum may obstruct breathing or interfere with the insertion of a nasogastric tube.

Nursing Diagnosis

Assessment data may reveal the following diagnosis:
- Knowledge deficit related to misinformation regarding use of over-the-counter nasal sprays.

Client Teaching

- Caution clients against overuse of over-the-counter nasal sprays.
- Instruct parents on care of children with nosebleeds: Have the child sit up and lean forward to avoid aspiration of blood; apply pressure to the anterior of nose with thumb and forefinger as the child breathes through mouth; apply ice or cold cloth over bridge of nose if pressure fails to stop bleeding.
- Elderly people lose the sense of smell and thus should have smoke detectors in their homes.

Mouth and Pharynx

15

The nurse's assessment of the oral cavity determines the client's ability to masticate, salivate, and swallow. The condition of the oral cavity is also an important indication of a client's hygiene habits. The nurse examines the oral cavity for the presence of local or systemic changes that can interfere with a client's nutritional intake and predispose the client to more serious health alterations. Assessment may occur during administration of oral hygiene.

Anatomy and Physiology

The oral cavity is the anterior end of the digestive tract. Bordered by the lips, the entrance of the digestive tract leads to the oral cavity, which contains the teeth and gums, buccal mucosa, tongue, hard and soft palate, uvula, palatine tonsils, and pharynx (Fig. 19).

Rationale

The nurse inspects the mouth and pharynx to (1) detect signs of overall health status, (2) determine oral hygiene needs, and (3) develop care plans for clients with dehydration, restricted intake, facial trauma, or oral airway obstruction or who will undergo or have recently undergone surgery.

Mouth and Pharynx Assessment
Special Equipment

Penlight
Tongue depressor
Gauze square
Clean gloves to palpate any lesions

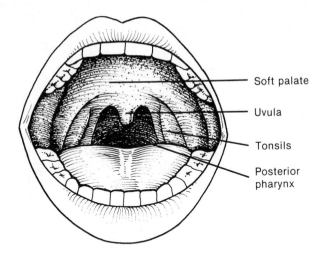

Fig. 19
Oral cavity.

Client Preparation

- Client may sit or lie.
- Ask the client to remove dentures and retainers.

History

- Determine whether dentures or retainers the client wears are comfortable.
- Has the client had a recent change in appetite or weight?
- Assess the client's dental hygiene practices and determine when the client last visited a dentist.
- Does the client smoke or chew tobacco; these habits increase the risk of mouth and throat cancer.
- Does the client have any pain or lesions of the mouth?

Assessment Techniques

Assessment	Normal Findings
Inspect lips for color, texture, hydration, contour, and lesions.	Pink, moist, symmetric, smooth.

Assessment	Normal Findings
Retract lips with gloved fingers, tongue depressor, or gauze; inspect mucosa for color, texture, hydration, and lesions.	Glistening pink; hyperpigmentation normal in 10% of Caucasians and 90% of blacks older than 50 years of age.
Inspect buccal mucosa by retracting cheek with a gloved finger or tongue depressor. Use a penlight to view posterior mucosa.	Mucosa is glistening pink, soft, and moist.
If lesions are present palpate them with gloved hand.	No lesions present.
Inspect gums for color, edema, retraction, bleeding, and lesions. Palpate gums for firmness.	Pink, moist, smooth.
Inspect teeth for dental hygiene needs, presence of dental caries, extraction sites, and color.	Smooth, white, shiny.
Note number of teeth.	Normal adults have 32 teeth.
Use a tongue depressor to view molars.	
Have the client relax mouth and protrude tongue halfway. Inspect for color, size, texture, position, presence of lesions or coating.	Medium red or pink, moist, slightly rough on top surface and smooth along lateral margins.
Have the client raise tongue and move it side to side.	Moves freely.
Take care to view undersurface of tongue and floor of mouth for color and lesions.	Pink and moist.
Palpate sides and base of the tongue and the floor of the mouth with gloved fingers for lesions.	Smooth and without lesions.

Assessment	Normal Findings
Have the client tip head back and hold mouth open so that the nurse can inspect hard and soft palates for color, shape, texture, and extra bony prominences or defects.	Light pink, soft palate is smooth. Hard palate is rough. Bony growth between the two palates is common.
Explain pharynx examination to the client. Tip head back, open mouth, say "ah" with tongue depressor on middle third of tongue; using penlight inspect for inflammation, lesions, edema, petechiae, exudate.	Pink and well-hydrated. Clear exudate found with chronic sinus problems.
Note landmarks of tonsillar pillars, uvula, soft palate, and posterior pharynx.	Uvula and soft palate rise as client says "ah."

Deviations from Normal 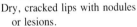	Nurse Alert
Dry, cracked lips with nodules or lesions.	
Thick white patches (leukoplakia) on mucosa, gums, or tongue.	Could be a precancerous sign. Also seen in heavy smokers and alcoholics.
Spongy gums that bleed easily indicate periodontal disease.	
In teeth: chalky white discoloration (indicates early caries) or brown/black discoloration (advanced caries).	
In pharynx: edema, petechiae, lesions; yellow/green exudate indicates infection; reddened edematous uvula and tonsillar pillars indicate inflammation.	

Nursing Diagnosis

Assessment data may reveal the following nursing diagnoses:

- Altered oral mucous membrane related to poor hygiene and chronic tobacco use.
- Pain related to inflammation of oral mucosa.
- Knowledge deficit regarding oral hygiene related to misinformation.
- Potential for infection related to poor oral hygiene practices.
- Altered health maintenance related to lack of knowledge.

Pediatric Considerations

- Children have 20 deciduous teeth that erupt between 8 to 30 months of age depending on the tooth. Permanent teeth begin to appear around 6 years of age with final molars in place at 12 to 17 years of age.

Gerontologic Considerations

- In elderly people, the mucosa is normally dry because of reduced salivation and the gums are pale.
- An elderly person's teeth often feel rough when tooth enamel calcifies. Yellow or darkened teeth are also common.

Client Teaching

- Discuss proper techniques for oral hygiene, including brushing and flossing.
- Explain early warning signs of oral cancer including a sore in the mouth that bleeds easily and does not heal in 2 to 3 weeks, a lump or thickening in the mouth, numbness or pain in mouth and throat, and red or white patches on mucosa that persist.
- Explain warning signs of gum (periodontal) disease, including gums that bleed easily, red, swollen gums that pull away from teeth, pus between teeth or around a loose tooth.
- Encourage yearly dental examinations for children and adults. Elderly people should visit a dentist every 6 months.
- Elderly clients should eat soft foods and cut food into small pieces because of difficulty in chewing.
- Warn parents not to put a child asleep with a bottle containing formula, milk, or juice, since these liquids may pool and cause tooth decay.

Neck

16

Assessment of the neck includes assessing the neck muscles, lymph nodes, thyroid gland, and trachea. The assessment of the carotid arteries and jugular veins is described in the section on the vascular system.

Anatomy and Physiology

The lymph nodes collect drainage of lymphatic fluid from the head and neck areas. Fig. 20 shows the location of major lymphatic chains in the head and neck. The thyroid gland lies in the anterior lower neck to both sides of the trachea, with the isthmus of the gland overlying the trachea. The trachea is located midline above the suprasternal notch. Fig. 21 shows the normal anatomic locations.

Rationale

The nurse inspects the neck for asymmetry, edema, masses, or scars. If any masses are seen, they should be palpated to determine size, shape, tenderness, consistency, and mobility.

Neck Assessment
Special Equipment

Stethoscope

Client Preparation

Ask the client to sit, raise the chin, and tilt the head back. Palpate the lymph nodes from behind or to the client's side. Palpate the thyroid gland from either the front or behind (client should lower the head to relax the neck muscles if palpated from behind).

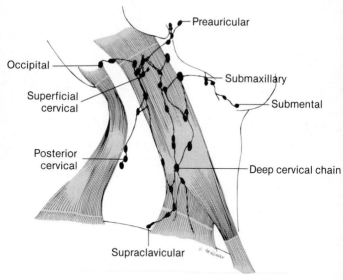

Fig. 20
Head and neck lymphatic chains.

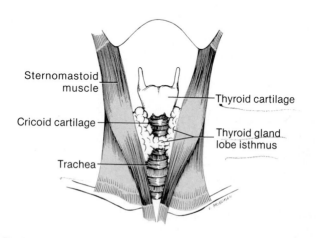

Fig. 21
Thyroid gland.

History

- Has the client had a recent cold or infection?
- Does the client have a history of thyroid problems or receiving thyroid medications?
- Does the client have neck pain or swelling?
- Review the client's history of pneumothorax or bronchial tumors, which can displace the trachea.

Assessment Techniques

Assessment	Normal Findings
Ask the client to flex the neck with the chin to the chest, hyperextend the neck backward, and move the head laterally to each side and then sideways so that the ear moves toward the shoulder. This tests the sternocleidomastoid and trapezius muscles.	Moves freely, full range without discomfort: Flexion = 45 degrees Extension = 55 degrees Lateral abduction = 40 degrees
With the client's chin raised and head tilted back inspect the neck for asymmetry, edema, masses, or scars. Palpate any masses for size, shape, tenderness, consistency, and mobility.	The neck is normally symmetric without obvious masses.
Inspect the lymph node areas and compare both sides. Inspect the lower neck over the thyroid gland for masses and symmetry.	Nodes are not visible.
Ask the client to extend the neck and swallow; note any bulging of the thyroid gland.	The thyroid gland cannot be visualized on swallowing.
Have the client relax with neck flexed slightly forward or toward side of the examiner to relax tissues and muscles.	Normally lymph nodes are not easily palpable.

Assessment	Normal Findings
Use the pads of the middle three fingers and palpate each lymph node in a rotary motion. Check each node methodically and compare both sides of the neck. Assess for size, shape, delineation, mobility, consistency, and tenderness.	Small (less than 1 cm), mobile, soft, nontender nodes are not uncommon.
To palpate the thyroid gland by the posterior approach have the client lower the chin and place both hands around the client's neck with fingertips over the lower trachea.	
Palpate the isthmus on swallowing.	The thyroid isthmus is more easily palpated than the lobes, which lie behind the sternocleidomastoid muscle.
Palpate each lobe with the head turned slightly toward the side being examined (Fig. 22).	
Gently displace the lobe with one hand while palpating with the other.	
Ask the client to swallow.	The thyroid gland is more easily palpated in very thin clients. When palpable, the thyroid gland rises on swallowing.
If the thyroid appears enlarged, place the diaphragm of a stethoscope over the thyroid.	Normally no sound is heard.
Listen for vascular sounds.	
Palpate the trachea for position by slipping thumb and index finger to each side at the suprasternal notch.	The trachea is midline at the suprasternal notch.

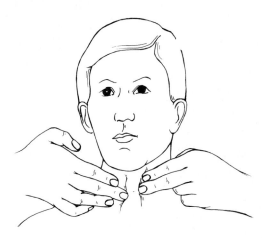

Fig. 22
Posterior approach for palpation of thyroid gland.

Deviations from Normal	Nurse Alert	

Asymmetric head position with rigid neck movement or reduced range of motion.

Lymph node enlargement may indicate localized or systemic infection.

Enlargement of the thyroid gland may indicate thyroid dysfunction or tumor.

Lateral displacement of the trachea may result from a mass in the neck or mediastinum or pulmonary abnormality.

Lymph nodes are sometimes permanently enlarged after serious infection; such enlarged nodes are usually nontender.

Malignant tumors in lymph nodes are usually hard, immobile, irregularly shaped, and nontender.

Masses or nodules in the thyroid gland may indicate malignancy.

Nursing Diagnosis

Assessment data may reveal the following diagnosis:
- Impaired physical mobility related to neck pain or muscle stiffness.

Pediatric Considerations

Children may normally have moderate number of small, firm lymph nodes.

Gerontologic Considerations

Elderly clients may have reduced range of motion in neck resulting from arthritic changes.

Client Teaching

- Stress the importance of regular compliance with medication schedule to clients with thyroid disease.
- Instruct the client to call a physician if an enlarged lump or mass is noted in neck.

Thorax and Lungs

17

Examination of the thorax and lungs involves the assessment of three areas: the posterior thorax, the lateral thorax, and the anterior thorax, described separately in the following sections.

Anatomy and Physiology

The two primary physiologic functions of the lungs are oxygenation of the blood and maintenance of acid-base balance. Altered lung function can thus affect other body systems.

During assessment, keep in mind the underlying position of the lungs (Fig. 23) and the position of each rib. Anteriorly, count the intercostal spaces from the second rib extending from the angle of Louis. Posteriorly, identify intercostal spaces from the seventh rib at the level of the inferior margin of the scapula. From there count upward to locate the third thoracic vertebrate and align with inner borders of the scapula. The spinous process of the third thoracic vertebrate and the fourth, fifth, and sixth ribs helps to locate the lung's lateral lobes. Anatomic landmarks must be used for an accurate assessment (Fig. 24).

Rationale

Pulmonary disease can be acute or chronic, and nurses in all settings can screen clients early for disorders and assess long-term disabilities. This assessment is particularly important for clients at risk for developing pulmonary complications, including clients for whom bed rest is prescribed or clients with chest or abdominal pain impairing deep breathing.

Thorax and Lung Assessment
Special Equipment

Stethoscope

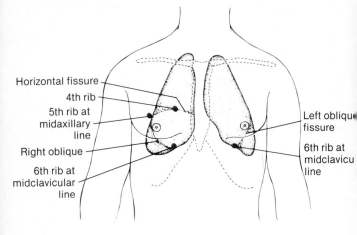

Horizontal fissure
4th rib
5th rib at midaxillary line
Right oblique
6th rib at midclavicular line
Left oblique fissure
6th rib at midclavicular line

Fig. 23
Anterior position of lung lobes in relation to anatomic landmarks.
(From Potter PA and Perry AG: Fundamentals, of nursing: concepts, process, and practice, ed 2, St Louis, 1989. The CV Mosby Co.)

Client Preparation

- Client must be undressed to the waist.
- Make sure lighting is good.
- Client sits for assessment of posterior and lateral chest. Client may sit or lie for assessment of anterior chest.

History

- Assess history of smoking, including number of years smoked, cigarettes or cigars smoked per day, and amount of pipe smoking.
- Does the client have a cough (productive or nonproductive), sputum production, shortness of breath, orthopnea, and poor activity tolerance?
- Does the client work in an environment that contains pollutants?
- Assess history of allergies to pollens, dust, or other airborne irritants, as well as to foods, drugs, or chemical substances.
- Review the client's family history for cancer, tuberculosis, allergies, and chronic obstructive pulmonary disease, for example asthma and emphysema.

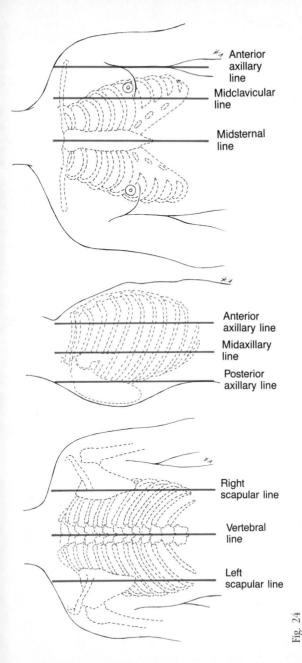

Fig. 24

Anatomic chest wall landmarks. **A,** Posterior chest. **B,** Anterior chest. **C,** Lateral chest.
(From Potter PA and Perry AG: Fundamentals of nursing: concepts, process, and practice, ed 2, St Louis, 1989, The CV Mosby Co.)

Anterior
axillary
line

Midclavicular
line

Midsternal
line

Anterior
axillary
line

Midaxillary
line

Posterior
axillary
line

Right
scapular
line

Vertebral
line

Left
scapular
line

Assessment Techniques
Posterior thorax

Assessment	Normal Findings
Observe for any signs or symptoms in other body systems that may indicate pulmonary problems. Reduced oxygenation can cause, for example, reduced mental alertness or signs of cyanosis in the skin or mucous membranes.	
Observe the shape of the chest. Note the anterior-posterior diameter.	Chest contour is symmetric and anterior-posterior diameter is normally twice as wide as chest is deep (almost round in infants).
Observe for bulging of the intercostal spaces on expiration.	No bulging or active movement should occur in the intercostal spaces with breathing.
Note position of spine, slope of ribs, and symmetry of scapula.	Spine is normally straight without lateral deviation. Scapulae are symmetric and closely attached to chest wall. Posteriorly ribs slope across and down.
Observe the thorax as a whole.	Normally expands and relaxes with equality of movement bilaterally.
Palpate the posterior thorax for lumps, masses, or tenderness; with pain or tenderness, avoid deep palpation because fractured rib fragments may displace against vital organs.	Palpation is painless if no masses are present.

Assessment	Normal Findings
Measure chest excursion:	
Stand behind the client and place the hands parallel over lower portion of rib cage on both sides of the spine.	
The fingers should be about 2 inches (5 cm) apart, with thumbs pointing toward the spine and fingers pointing laterally.	
Press hands (do not slide) toward spine to create a small skinfold between the thumbs.	
After exhalation ask the client to take a deep breath and observe the movement of your thumbs.	Chest excursion should separate the thumbs 1½ to 2 inches (3 to 5 cm).
During chest excursion palpate for symmetry of respiration.	Chest movement is symmetric.
Palpate for tactile (vocal) fremitus:	
Place the ball or lower palm of hand on symmetric areas of thorax, beginning at the lung apex (Fig. 25)	Tactile fremitus is symmetric and strongest at top near the tracheal bifurcation and decreases over periphery of chest
At each position ask client to say "99."	
If fremitus is faint, ask client to speak louder or in a lower tone.	Normally a faint vibration is felt.
Percuss the chest wall to determine whether lung tissue is air filled, fluid filled, or solid:	

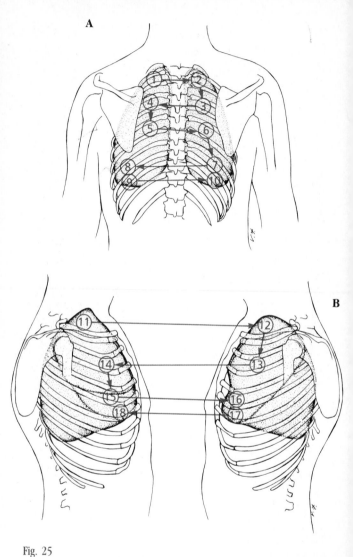

Fig. 25
A to **C,** The nurse follows systematic pattern when comparing fremitus, percussion, and auscultation.
(From Potter PA and Perry AG: Fundamentals of nursing: concepts, process, and practice, ed 2, St Louis, 1989, The CV Mosby Co.)

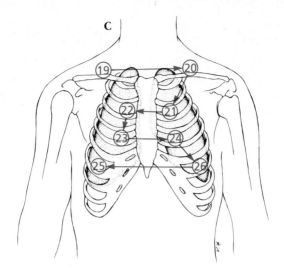

Fig. 25, **C**.
For legend see opposite page.

Assessment	Normal Findings
Ask the client to fold arms across chest.	
With indirect percussion technique, percuss intercostal spaces following a systematic pattern to compare both sides (Fig. 26).	The posterior thorax is normally resonant on percussion. Percussion over scapula, ribs, or spine is dull.
Auscultate lung sounds to detect mucus or obstructed airways and the lung's condition: Use the stethoscope diaphragm for adults and the bell for children. Place stethoscope over intercostal spaces. Ask the client to breathe slowly and deeply with the mouth slightly open.	Normal breath sounds include bronchovesicular sounds between the scapula (a blowing sound with equal inspiratory and expiratory phases) and vesicular sounds at the lungs' periphery (soft, breezy, low-pitched sounds, with the inspiratory phase lasting about three times longer than the expiratory phase).

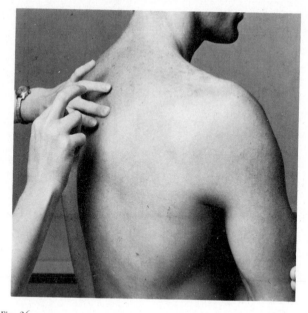

Fig. 26
Position of client for percussion of posterior of chest wall.
(From Potter PA and Perry AG: Fundamentals of nursing: concepts, process, and practice, ed 2, St Louis, 1989, The CV Mosby Co.)

Assessment	Normal Findings
Listen to full inspiration and expiration at each position. Follow the same systematic pattern as with percussion to compare both sides.	

Assessment	Normal Findings
If tactile fremitus, percussion, or auscultation reveals abnormalities, auscultate for altered voice sounds with stethoscope placed over same locations to hear breath sounds. Have the client say "99" or whisper "one, two, three"	In bronchophony, the "99" is normally muffled and whispered pectoriloquy sounds are muffled.

Deviations from Normal	Nurse Alert
Abnormal chest contours may be caused by congenital and postural alterations and aging.	
A barrel chest may indicate chronic lung disease.	
Bulging in the intercostal spaces indicates labored breathing.	
Palpate any mass or swollen area for size, shape, and qualities of a lesion.	Avoid deep palpation to avoid risk of displacing fractured rib fragments against vital organs.
Reduced chest excursion may be caused by pain, postural deformity, or fatigue.	
Reduced tactile fremitus may indicate accumulations of mucus, collapsed lung tissue, or lung lesions.	
Dull percussion notes indicate underlying bone or fluid-filled lung.	
Flat percussion notes may indicate a lung mass.	

Deviations from Normal	Nurse Alert
Adventitious (abnormal) breath sounds include crackles (rales), rhonchi, wheezes, and pleural friction rub (Table 12).	
The absence of lung sounds may indicate collapsed lung or surgically removed lobes.	

Lateral thorax

Assessment	Normal Findings
With client remaining seated and arms raised above the head, extend assessment to lateral thorax.	
Inspect, palpate, percuss, and auscultate lateral thorax in same manner as with posterior thorax.	Percussion notes are resonant. Breath sounds are vesicular.
Use a systematic method to compare both sides.	Excursion cannot be assessed laterally.

Deviations from Normal
Same as with posterior thorax.

Anterior thorax

Assessment	Normal Findings
With client seated, observe the accessory muscles of breathing: sternomastoid, trapezius, and abdominal muscles.	The accessory muscles move little with normal passive breathing.
Observe the costal angle.	The angle is usually larger than 90 degrees between the two costal margins.

Table 12 Adventitious sounds

Sound	Site auscultated	Cause	Character
Crackles (rales) fine or course	Most common in dependent lobes: right and left lung bases	Random sudden reinflation of groups of alveoli	Sound like crackling; heard usually during inspiration; vary in pitch: high, medium, or low; often cleared by coughing
Rhonchi	Primarily over trachea and bronchi; if loud enough, intensity can be heard over majority of lung fields	Fluid located in larger airways causing more turbulence	Sound like coarse rattling; heard more during expiration; louder and lower pitched than rales; may be cleared by coughing
Wheezes	Can be heard over all lung fields	Narrowed airways, that is, bronchospasm	High-pitched, continuous musical sound heard during inspiration or expiration; does not clear with coughing
Pleural friction rub	Anterior lateral lung field (if client sits upright)	Pleura becomes inflamed; parietal pleura rubs against visceral pleura	Has a grating quality; heard best on inspiration; does not clear with coughing

Assessment	Normal Findings
Assess respiratory rate and rhythm (see Chapter 8). Palpate for masses or tenderness.	Respiration of males is more diaphragmatic (more movement of abdominal muscles) and respiration of females is more costal (more movement of ribs).
Measure chest excursion: Place hands parallel on lateral rib cage with thumbs 2.5 inches (6 cm) apart and angled along each costal margin.	
Push thumbs toward midline to create a skinfold. Ask client to inhale deeply. Observe separation of thumbs.	Chest excursion should separate the thumbs 1½ to 2 inches (3 to 5 cm).
Palpate for tactile fremitus, using the same method as with the posterior thorax. With the client sitting or supine, percuss the anterior thorax comparing both sides, considering the locations of the underlying liver, heart, and stomach (Fig. 27).	Fremitus is normally decreased over the heart, lower thorax, and breast tissue. Percussion notes over the heart and liver are dull. The gastric air bubble is percussed as a tympanic sound.
Percuss in a systematic pattern from above the clavicles, moving across and down; displace female breasts as needed.	
With client sitting, auscultate the anterior thorax in the same pattern as with percussion. Pay particular attention to auscultating the lower lobes, where mucous secretions commonly accumulate.	Bronchovesicular and vesicular sounds are heard above and below the clavicles and along the lung periphery. Bronchial sounds are normal over the trachea: loud, high-pitched, and hollow sounding, with expiration lasting longer than inspiration.

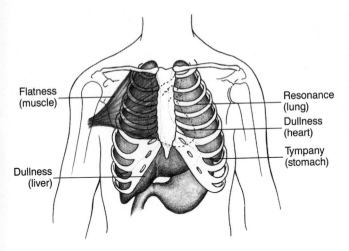

Flatness (muscle)

Resonance (lung)

Dullness (heart)

Tympany (stomach)

Dullness (liver)

Fig. 27
Variations in percussion notes in normal thorax and upper abdomen.
(From Potter PA and Perry AG: Fundamentals of nursing: concepts, process, and practice, ed 2, St Louis, 1989, The CV Mosby Co.)

Deviations from Normal

With difficult breathing, accessory muscles can be seen contracting. Clients with chronic obstructive pulmonary disease breathe noisily and may produce a grunting sound.
See deviations for posterior thorax.

Nursing Diagnoses

Assessment data may reveal the following diagnoses:
- Ineffective airway clearance related to tracheobronchial mucus obstruction.
- Ineffective breathing pattern related to pain.
- Impaired gas exchange related to altered oxygen supply.

Pediatric Considerations

In children younger than 6 years of age, ventilatory movement is mainly abdominal or diaphragmatic rather than costal. Infants have a thin chest wall with a bony and cartilaginous rib cage that is soft and pliant. Lungs are usually hyperresonant throughout in infants and young children. Breath sounds are louder and harsher.

Gerontologic Considerations

Because of calcification of the vertebral cartilages, reduced mobility of the ribs, partial contraction of the intercostal muscles, and kyphosis that frequently occurs with aging, older adults do not breathe as deeply as younger adults. An older client, particularly a bedridden client, may complain of discomfort and have difficulty coughing productively.

Client Teaching

- Explain risk factors for chronic obstructive lung disease and lung cancer, including cigarette smoking, history of smoking more than 20 years, and exposure to environmental pollution.
- Discuss warning signs of lung cancer, including persistent cough, sputum streaked with blood, chest pains, and recurrent attacks of pneumonia or bronchitis.
- Instruct clients with excessive mucus about deep breathing exercises, coughing, intake of fluids, postural drainage, and chest percussion.
- Instruct elderly clients regarding benefits of influenza and pneumonia vaccinations to reduce chances of respiratory infection.
- Refer interested clients to smoking cessation programs.

Heart and Vascular System

18

Assessment of the heart and vascular system should be performed together because alterations in either system may be manifest as changes in the other. If the nursing history reveals heart disease or the presence of risk factors such as smoking, alcohol consumption, and poor eating and exercise patterns, observe more carefully for abnormalities.

Heart
Anatomy and Physiology

The heart is located in the middle of the mediastinum, bounded on both sides by the lung. It is a pulsatile, four-chambered pump that delivers blood to the lung and the arterial system. Its unique electrical conduction system and contractile properties provide for regular rhythmic contractions to maintain an average cardiac output of 5 liters of blood per minute to vital tissues. The arterial system is a branching network of blood vessels that maintains a pressure necessary to deliver blood to distant peripheral tissues. The ability of the arterial system to compensate for changes in heart function, blood volume, and blood flow ensures the delivery of oxygen and nutrients to the body's cells.

Fig. 28 shows the normal position of the heart in the adult. The infant's and young child's heart is positioned more horizontally and has a relatively larger diameter. Heart displacement is common in older adults as a result of kyphosis and scoliosis.

To assess heart function the nurse must understand the cardiac cycle and the physiologic signs of each event.

The left heart sounds occur as follows in relation to the cardiac cycle:

The left ventricle fills through the mitral valve from the left atrium, and the mitral valve closes, causing the first heart sound (S_1).

151

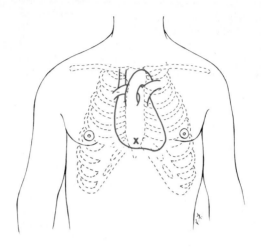

Fig. 28
Anatomic position of heart in relation to sternum and ribs.
(From Potter PA and Perry AG: Fundamentals of nursing: concepts, process, and practice, ed 2, St Louis, 1989, The CV Mosby Co.)

The ventricle contracts and blood flows through the aortic valve into the aorta. After the ventricle empties, the aortic valve closes, causing the second heart sound (S_2).

The mitral valve reopens for rapid ventricular filling, creating a third heart sound (S_3) that is heard more often in children and young adults.

The atrium contracts to enhance ventricular filling, producing the fourth heart sound (S_4), which is not normally heard in adults.

Rationale

Assessment of cardiovascular function involves a thorough evaluation of apical and peripheral pulses, the events that occur in relation to the cardiac cycle, and the overall integrity of the heart and major arteries. Heart disease is the leading cause of death in the United States and Canada. The nurse's assessment serves not only to detect cardiovascular alterations, but also to focus on potential problems the client can be educated to control or prevent.

Heart Assessment
Special equipment

Stethoscope

Client preparation

The client should lie supine with the upper body slightly elevated, and the examiner should stand at the client's right side. Ask the client not to talk during the assessment.

To avoid alarming clients do not show any concern about findings during assessment.

History

- Assess history of smoking, exercise habits, and dietary patterns including intake.
- Is the client taking medications for cardiovascular function? If so, does the client know their purpose, dosage, and side effects?
- Ask whether the client has chest pain, palpitations, excess fatigue, dyspnea, edema of feet, cyanosis, fainting, or orthopnea. Do symptoms occur during rest or exercise?
- Does the client have a stressful life-style?
- Assess the client's family history for heart disease or hypertension.
- Does the client have known heart disease including congestive heart failure, congenital heart disease, coronary artery disease, and cardiac dysrhythmia?

Assessment techniques

Assessment	Normal Findings	

Perform inspection and palpation together:

Locate landmarks of the chest, first by palpating the angle of Louis, or sternal angle, which is felt as a ridge in the sternum approximately 2 inches below the sternal notch. Skip the fingers along the angle on each side of the sternum to feel the adjacent second ribs.

Assessment	Normal Findings
The second intercostal space (ICS) is just below each rib.	
Inspect and palpate each anatomic landmark. Inspect for appearance of pulsations. View each area at an angle.	No pulsations are normally seen.
Palpate vibrations with the heel of the hand and pulsations with the fingertips.	

Inspect and palpate at:

Assessment	Normal Findings
1. Aortic area (right second ICS) (Fig. 29) 2. Pulmonic area (left second ICS) 3. Tricuspid area (left fifth ICS)	No vibrations or pulsations palpated in aortic, pulmonic, or tricuspid area.
4. Apical or mitral area (left fifth ICS at midclavicular line) Note if apical impulse can be palpated. This is the PMI. If apical impulse cannot be felt have client turn onto left side.	Normal apical impulse or point of maximal impulse (PMI). Is a light tap felt in an area 1 to 2 cm ($\frac{1}{2}$ inch) in diameter.
5. Epigastric area (just below tip of sternum)	Pulsation of abdominal aorta may be felt and seen.

Percussion:

Assessment	Normal Findings
For adults, percussion of heart borders to determine heart size is very difficult (x-ray films are preferred).	Heart is normally dull to percussion.
Percuss the infant's or young child's heart borders to determine size.	

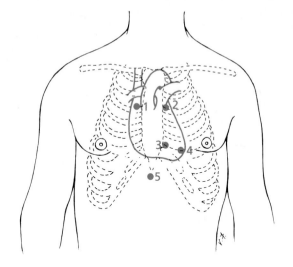

Fig. 29
Sites for assessment of cardiac function.
(From Potter PA and Perry, AG: Fundamentals of nursing: concepts, process, and practice, ed 2, St Louis, 1989, The CV Mosby Co.)

Assessment	Normal Findings
Auscultation is performed to detect normal heart sounds, extra heart sounds, and murmurs:	
Eliminate any room noise.	
If it takes several seconds to hear heart sounds, explain this to client to prevent concern.	
Lift a female client's left breast to hear over the chest wall better.	

Assessment	Normal Findings
Auscultate using the diaphragm of the stethoscope, since normal heart sounds are high pitched. Begin auscultating at the PMI, then move methodically and systematically to the tricuspid, pulmonic, and aortic areas. Hear both sounds clearly at each location. Then repeat the sequence with the bell of the stethoscope applied lightly to the chest.	S_1 is high pitched and dull in quality, sounds like "lub," and precedes the short systolic phase. Occurs at same time as carotid pulsation. S_2 is high pitched, sounds like "dub," and follows the short systolic phase. *Normal relative loudness of S_1 and S_2 are:* Apical area: S_1 at its loudest, louder than S_2. Tricuspid area: S_1 louder than S_2. Pulmonic area: S_2 louder than S_1. Aortic area: S_2 at its loudest, louder than S_1.
Assess heart rate: Each combination of S_1 and S_2 counts as one heartbeat.	Normal rate is 60 to 100 beats/min in an adult.
Assess heart rhythm: Note the time between S_1 and S_2 (systolic pause) and then the time between S_2 and the next S_1 (diastolic pause).	Regular rhythm involves intervals between each sequence of beats.
If heart rhythm is irregular, compare apical and radial pulse rates to determine whether a pulse deficit exists. Auscultate the apical pulse first and then immediately assess the radial pulse (one examiner). Compare the two rates simultaneously (two examiners).	If a deficit exists, the radial pulse is usually slower than the apical pulse.

Assessment	Normal Findings
Auscultate for extra heart sounds at each auscultatory site:	
Use bell of stethoscope and listen for low-pitched extra sounds S$_3$ and S$_4$.	S$_3$ occurs just after S$_2$, and S$_4$ occurs just before S$_1$. S$_3$ is commonly heard in children and young adults.
Auscultate for murmurs at each auscultatory site:	
Note timing, location, radiation, intensity, pitch, and quality.	Normally no murmurs are heard.
To assess for radiation listen over areas besides where it is heard best, such as the neck or back.	

Deviations from Normal	Nurse Alert
Sinus bradycardia: regular rhythm but decreased rate (40 to 60 beats per minute), common in well-conditioned athletes.	
Sinus tachycardia: regular rhythm but increased rate (more than 100 beats/min) common after exercise or caffeine or alcohol ingestion.	
Sinus dysrhythmia: pulse rate changes during respiration increasing at the peak of inspiration and declining during expiration.	
Ventricular premature contraction: results from abnormal electrical conduction. Heartbeat occurs out of rhythm.	

Deviations from Normal	Nurse Alert
With pulse deficits, the radial pulse is generally slower than the apical pulse.	Report any pulse deficit to the physician immediately.
Heart murmurs are recorded by intensity: Grade I: Barely audible Grade II: Audible immediately but faint Grade III: Loud without thrust or thrill Grade IV: Loud with thrust or thrill Grade V: Very loud with thrust or thrill; heard with stethoscope applied only lightly Grade VI: Louder; may be heard without stethoscope; quality is blowing, musical, harsh, or rumbling	

Nursing diagnoses

Assessment data may reveal the following nursing diagnoses:
- Decreased cardiac output related to conduction abnormality.
- Activity intolerance related to oxygen supply and demand imbalance.

Pediatric considerations

The point of maximal impulse (PMI) of an infant can usually be found near the third or fourth ICS at the midclavicular line. A child's thin chest wall makes it easy to palpate the PMI.

Gerontologic considerations

It may be difficult to locate the PMI, since the chest deepens in its anterior-posterior diameters.

Client teaching

- Explain risk factors for heart disease, including high dietary intake of cholesterol, lack of regular aerobic exercise, smoking, stressful life-style, and family history of heart disease. Obesity and excessive alcohol consumption may also be risks.
- Refer client (if appropriate) to resources for controlling or reducing risks (for example, nutritional counseling, exercise class, and stress reduction programs)
- For clients with heart disease explain the importance of compliance with the treatment program.
- Teach clients who take heart medication how to measure their own pulse.

Vascular System

Assessment of the vascular system includes measuring blood pressure (see Chapter 9) and assessing integrity of accessible arteries and veins.

The time for total physical assessment can be minimized by integrating vascular system assessment with the assessment of other body areas.

Anatomy and Physiology

When the left ventricle pumps blood into the aorta, pressure waves are transmitted throughout the arterial system. The carotid artery pulse reflects heart function. Both carotid arteries supply blood to the brain; however, occlusion of either can cause serious brain damage.

The most accessible veins to assess are the internal and external jugular. Both veins drain from the head and neck into the superior vena cava. The external jugular lies superficially and can be seen just above the clavicle. The internal jugular lies deeper, along the carotid artery.

The peripheral arteries deliver oxygenated blood to the extremities. Hand function is impaired by reduced circulation in the brachial artery but not necessarily by impairment of the radial or ulnar artery because of their interconnected circulation. Similarly, the foot is protected by interconnections between the posterior tibial and dorsalis pedis arteries.

Vascular Assessment
Special equipment

Stethoscope
Sphygmomanometer (for blood pressure measurement)
Ruler or tape measure in centimeters

Client preparation

- Client sits during examination of the carotid arteries.
- Client lies supine during assessment of the jugular veins and peripheral arteries and veins.

History

- Does the client experience leg cramps, numbness, tingling, pain in the feet or legs, or burning in the extremities?
- If leg pain or cramps are present, are they aggravated by walking or standing for long periods or during sleep?
- Does the client notice edema, coldness, or cyanosis in the legs or ankles?
- Ask whether the client wears tight garters or hosiery.
- Assess medical history for hypertension, phlebitis, diabetes, or varicose veins.

Assessment techniques
Carotid arteries

Assessment	Normal Findings
Assess the carotid arteries with the client seated:	
Examine only one carotid artery at a time. Do not vigorously palpate so that carotid sinus stimulation is avoided.	The carotid pulse is localized, strong, thrusting, and unchanged by inspiration, expiration, or position changes.
Inspect the neck for artery pulsation.	Both carotid arteries should be equal in pulse rate, rhythm, strength, and elasticity.
Ask the client to turn head slightly toward the side being examined.	
Palpate gently with index and middle fingers at medial edge of sternomastoid muscle (Fig. 30).	

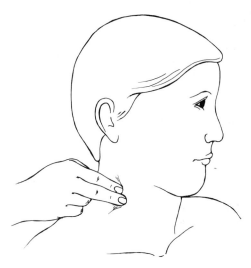

Fig. 30
Anatomic position of carotid artery.

Assessment	Normal Findings
Note the rate, rhythm, strength, and elasticity of pulse. Check opposite carotid pulse separately for symmetry.	Rate same as apical pulse, regular, strong, elastic, and equal.
Auscultate the carotid pulse as the client holds breath.	No sound is heard over the carotid arteries on auscultation.

Jugular veins

Assessment	Normal Findings
Assess the jugular veins for venous pressure:	
Ask the client to recline in a supine position with head raised about 30 degrees.	Normal veins are flat.

Assessment	Normal Findings
Be sure neck and upper thorax are exposed; do not flex or hyperextend neck. If jugular vein is visible, determine the highest visible point of the jugular vein.	
Measure the venous pressure as the vertical distance in inches (centimeters) between the point of jugular distention and the sternal angle or suprasternal notch. Repeat the same measurement on the other side.	Venous pressure is 1½ inches (3-4 cm) or less.

Blood pressure

Assessment	Normal Findings
Assess the client's blood pressure in both arms, auscultating brachial arteries (see Chapter 9).	Difference of 5 to 10 mm Hg between the two arms.

Peripheral circulation

Assessment	Normal Findings
Assess the skin, nail beds, and extremities for signs of venous or arterial insufficiency: color, temperature, pulse, edema, sensation, and skin changes.	Color is same as normal skin; skin is warm. The client can identify light and deep touch (see Chapter 24).

Table 13   Classification of pulse strength

Pulse Classification	Characteristics
0	No pulse palpable.
1+	Pulse is difficult to palpate, weak and thready in character, and easy to obliterate.
2+	Pulse is difficult to palpate, and light pressure will locate pulse. Discriminating touch senses it is stronger than 1.
3+	Pulse is normal, easy to palpate, and not easily obliterated.
4+	Pulse is strong, easy to palpate, seems to bound against fingertips, and cannot be obliterated.

Assessment	Normal Findings

Palpate each peripheral artery for:

Elasticity of vessel wall.
Pulse rate, rhythm, strength (see Table 13), and equality.
Palpate the radial pulse lightly along radial groove (Fig. 31) at the wrist.
Palpate the ulnar pulse (Fig. 32) if arterial insufficiency to the hand is suspected. Pulse is on ulnar side of wrist.

Peripheral pulses are normally easy to palpate, with vessel walls elastic, rhythm regular, and rate within normal range for client's age.

Nurse Alert

If radial and ulnar pulses are weak, perform an Allen test:
Have the client make a fist.
Compare ulnar and radial arteries simultaneously.
Ask the client to open hand.
Release ulnar artery.
Observe whether hand turns pink to reveal adequate collateral circulation. (Examiners may repeat by releasing radial artery.)

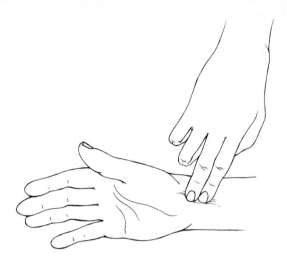

Fig. 31
Anatomic position of radial artery.

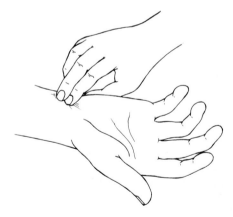

Fig. 32
Anatomic position of ulnar artery.

Assessment	Normal Findings

With the client's arm extended, palpate the brachial pulse in the groove between the biceps and triceps muscles at the antecubital fossa (Fig. 33).

Palpate the femoral pulse with the client supine (Fig. 34); the pulse is located midway between the symphysis pubis and the anterosuperior iliac spine; deep or bimanual (hands on both sides of the pulse site) palpation may be required.

Palpate popliteal pulse behind the knee (Fig. 35) with client prone or supine with slightly flexed knee, foot resting on the examination table, and leg muscles relaxed.

Palpate the dorsalis pedis pulse (Fig. 36) on the upper aspect of foot along an imaginary line extending from groove formed between big and second toe (may be congenitally absent).

Palpate posterior tibial pulse (Fig. 37) just below lateral malleolus with foot relaxed and slightly extended.

Assess status of peripheral veins

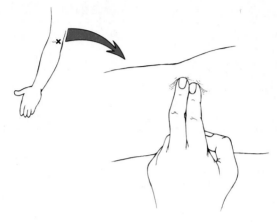

Fig. 33
Anatomic position of brachial artery.

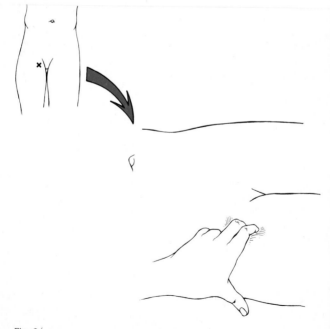

Fig. 34
Anatomic position of femoral artery.

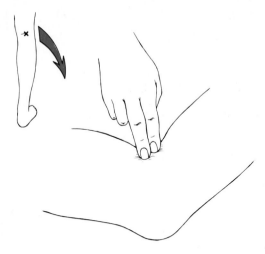

Fig. 35
Anatomic position of popliteal artery.

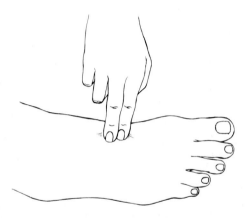

Fig. 36
Anatomic position of dorsalis pedis artery.

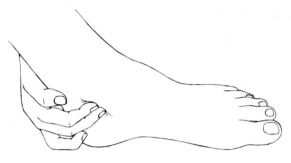

Fig. 37
Anatomic position of posterior tibial artery.

Assessment	Normal Findings
Inspect the lower extremities for varicosities (swollen or tortuous veins), peripheral edema, and phlebitis.	Veins normally are not visible. Small spiderlike capillaries visible along thigh are normal.
Assess for pitting edema around the ankles. Press the thumb firmly for at least 5 seconds over each medial malleolus or each shin.	No permanent depression left in the skin.
Assess for deep vein phlebitis by looking for a Homans' sign: extend client's leg and dorsiflex the foot. Inspect and palpate calves for localized redness, tenderness, and swelling over vein sites.	No calf soreness or pain. Color same as normal skin color without tenderness.
Assess further for deep phlebitis by quickly squeezing calf muscle against the tibia.	No calf pain.

Deviations from Normal	Nurse Alert
Narrowing of the carotid artery lumen may result in blood flow disturbances heard as blowing (bruit) or swishing sounds on auscultation.	Be very careful in palpating the carotid arteries to prevent stimulation of the carotid sinus, producing a drop in heart rate and blood pressure.
Elevated venous pressure (above 1½ inches [3 cm]) is a sign of heart disease.	
Impaired circulation to the extremities may be caused by systemic diseases, such as arteriosclerosis, atherosclerosis, and diabetes, coagulation disorders, such as thrombosis and embolus, local trauma and surgery, such as contusion, fracture, and vascular surgery, or application of constricting devices, such as casts, dressings, elastic bandages, and restraints.	Do not continuously massage a tender or painful calf; it is felt that this increases risk of an embolus.

Signs of venous insufficiency in the extremities:
  Normal or cyanotic color
  Normal temperature
  Normal pulse
  Often marked edema
  Brown pigmentation around
    ankles

Signs of arterial insufficiency in the extremities:
  Pale color on elevation,
  dusk red color when lowered.

Deviations from Normal	Nurse Alert

*Signs of arterial insufficiency
in the extremities:*

Cool temperature.
Decreased or absent pulse.
No edema or mild edema.
Shiny skin, decreased hair
growth.
Thickened nails.

A strong pulse may be caused
by exercise, fever, or emotional stress.

Inequality of pulses may indicate a local obstruction or
abnormal artery position.

A positive Homans' sign as
marked by pain or soreness
in the calves.

A permanent depression left in
the skin over the ankle following palpation reveals
edema. Measure depth of
the depression:

1 cm = 1+ edema
2 cm = 2+ edema
3 cm = 3+ edema
4 cm = 4+ edema

Nursing diagnoses

Assessment data may reveal the following nursing diagnoses:

- Potential activity intolerance related to impaired circulation to extremities.
- Altered peripheral tissue perfusion related to interrupted arteriovenous flow.

Pediatric considerations

- Absence of femoral pulse can be a sign of coarctation of the aorta.

Gerontologic considerations

- Auscultation of the carotid artery is especially important for clients in whom cerebrovascular disease is suspected.
- Dependent edema of the lower extremities is common in elderly clients.

Client teaching

- Tell clients their blood pressure reading. Explain normal readings for the client's age and implications of any abnormalities.
- Instruct clients with risk or evidence of vascular insufficiency in the lower extremities to avoid tight clothing over the lower body or legs; avoid sitting or standing for long periods, avoid crossing legs, walk regularly, and elevate feet when sitting.
- Elderly clients with hypertension may benefit from regular monitoring of blood pressure. Home monitoring kits are available. Teach clients how to use them.

Breasts

19

Anatomy and Physiology

The breasts of the female adult client normally extend in an area from the third to the sixth ribs. Each breast consists of glandular tissue, fat, and supportive fibrous ligaments (Fig. 38). An extensive series of lymphatic vessels and channels drain lymph from the breast into the axillary, supraclavicular, and infraclavicular nodes.

Rationale

The major role the nurse plays in assessing the breasts is to educate women about breast cancer and to screen for the presence of masses or irregularities in breast tissue. Because the breasts are associated with reproduction and a woman's sexuality, a high level of anxiety may be expressed by the client during an examination. Diseases of the breast also occur in men, and thus it is important to not overlook this portion of the examination in a male client.

Breast Assessment
Special Equipment

Small pillow

Client Preparation

Initially the client may sit or stand with arms at side. Remove gown for simultaneous viewing of both breasts. Optionally use a mirror to assist the woman in learning how to perform a self-examination.

During palpation have client sit and then lie supine with small pillow placed under upper back.

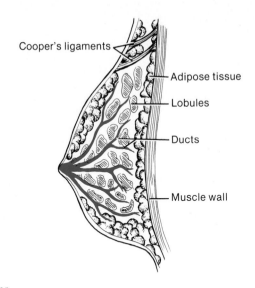

Fig. 38
Cross section of breast tissue.

History

- If a woman client is older than 50 years of age, determine whether she has a family history of breast cancer, had previous breast cancer, never had children, had a first child after age 30, or did not breastfeed any children (risk factors for breast cancer).
- Ask whether client (both sexes) has noticed pain or tenderness of breast, discharge from nipple, change in size of breast, or presence of a lump or mass. Have the client point out any masses.
- Ask the female client whether she performs a monthly breast self-examination. If so, determine time of month she performs it in relation to her menstrual cycle.
- Assess client's age at menarche, menopause, and first pregnancy (risk of cancer greatest in women who reach menarche before 13 years of age and have menopause after 50 years of age).
- Does client take oral contraceptives, digitalis, diuretics, steroids, or estrogen?

Assessment Techniques

Female Breast Assessment	Normal Findings
Inspect the size and symmetry of the breasts.	The breasts normally extend approximately from the third to the sixth ribs, with the nipple at the level of the fourth intercostal space.
Inspect the contour and shape of the breasts and note any masses or flattening.	
Inspect for retractions by asking client to raise arms over head, press hands against hips, and extend arms straight ahead while leaning forward.	Normal areola and nipple of Caucasians are pink (turning brown during pregnancy); in dark-skinned clients the areola and nipple are darker than other skin.
Inspect overlying skin for color, venous patterns, and presence of edema or inflammation.	Slight asymmetry in areola and nipples is not unusual.
Inspect nipple and areola for size and shape and the direction nipples point.	Breasts are smooth, round, and pendulous.
Note any discharge from the nipples.	No discharge normally; clear yellow discharge 2 days after childbirth is common.
If a client has large breasts, inspect undersurface carefully.	Skin smooth and dry.
	Normal developmental changes in the breasts include:
	Puberty: breast buds appear, nipples darken, areola diameter increases, and one breast may grow more rapidly.
	Young adulthood: breasts reach full normal size, shape is usually symmetric, and one breast may be larger.

Female Breast Assessment	Normal Findings

Pregnancy: breasts enlarge to two to three times their normal size, nipples enlarge and may become erect, areola darkens, superficial veins in the breasts become prominent, and a yellowish fluid (colostrum) may be expelled from the nipples.

Menopause: breasts shrink and tissue becomes softer, and sometimes it becomes flabby.

Older adult: chronic cystic disease diminishes after menopause. Adipose tissue increases, glandular tissue atrophies, suspensory ligaments relax, and breasts appear elongated or pendulous. Nipples become smaller.

Palpate lymph nodes with client sitting:

With a female client's arms at her sides, ask her to relax her muscles. Face the client and support her arm while abducting that same arm from the chest wall.

Place your hand against the client's chest wall and high in the axilla. With the fingertips press gently down over the surface of the ribs and muscles (Fig. 39).

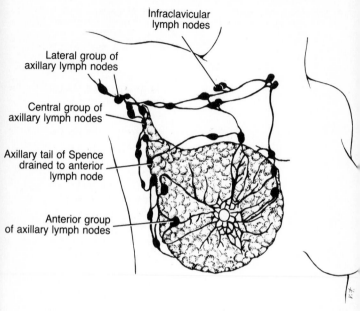

Fig. 39

Anatomic position of axillary and clavicular lymph nodes.
(From Potter PA and Perry AG: Fundamentals of nursing: concepts, process, and practice, ed 2, St Louis, 1989, The CV Mosby Co.)

Female Breast Assessment	Normal Findings
Palpate axillary nodes in four areas:	
Edge of pectoralis major along anterior axillary line.	
Chest wall in midaxillary area.	Lymph nodes are normally not palpable.
Upper part of humerus.	
Anterior edge of latissimus dorsi along posterior axillary line.	

Female Breast Assessment	Normal Findings
Palpate for supraclavicular and infraclavicular nodes.	
Palpate breast tissue with client supine and hands behind the neck; you may place small pillow under back.	
If client complains of a mass, begin with opposite breast for objective comparison.	The inframammary ridge at lower edge of each breast may feel firm or hard but should not be confused with a tumor.
With pads of first three fingers compress breast tissue gently against the chest wall (Fig. 40).	Breast tissue normally feels elastic. In fibrocystic disease, a common problem in women, tissue feels rather lumpy, but it is found bilaterally.
Palpate with circular motion, moving systematically along each quadrant and the tail (Fig. 41).	
Give greater attention to any areas of tenderness.	
Support large breasts with one hand and palpate breast tissue with the other against the supporting hand.	
Note consistency of tissues.	
Palpate any abnormal mass and record:	
Quadrant location (upper outer, lower outer, and so forth).	
Diameter.	
Shape (round, discoid, irregular).	
Consistency.	
Tenderness.	
Mobility.	
Discreteness (clear or unclear borders).	

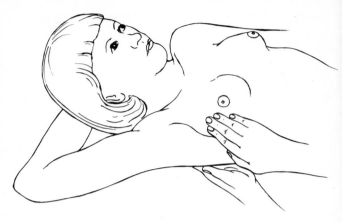

Fig. 40
Nurse palpates each breast quadrant using rotary motion of fingertips.

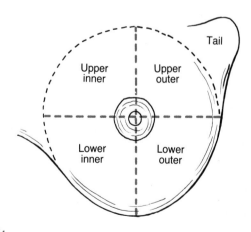

Fig. 41
Divide each breast into four quadrants and an axillary tail.
(From Potter PA and Perry AG: Fundamentals of nursing: concepts, process, and practice, ed 2, St Louis, 1989, The CV Mosby Co.)

Female Breast Assessment	Normal Findings
Palpate nipple and areola. Gently compress the nipple and note any discharge.	During examination, the nipple may normally become erect and the areola wrinkled.

Male Breast Assessment	Normal Findings
Inspect nipple and areola for nodules, edema, and ulceration. Palpate breast for same characteristics as with female breasts.	Enlarged male breast is caused by obesity or glandular enlargement.

Deviations from Normal	Nurse Alert
Difference in breast size may be normal or caused by inflammation or a mass. Rashes, ulcerations, bleeding, erythema, or discharge from nipples is abnormal. A palpable lymph node may be hard, tender, and immobile. *For males:* the same deviations may be present; the smaller amount of breast tissue in males presents lower risk of deviations.	Inverted or turned inward nipples may indicate an underlying growth. Retraction or dimpling may result from tumorous invasion of underlying ligaments. Cancerous lesions are generally hard, fixed, nontender, and irregularly shaped.

Nursing Diagnosis

Assessment data may reveal the following nursing diagnoses:

- Anxiety related to threat of cancer.
- Knowledge deficit regarding self-examination of breast related to inexperience.
- Impaired skin integrity related to ulceration.

Pediatric Considerations

See variations in inspection.

Gerontologic Considerations

See variations in inspection.

Client Teaching

- Women should perform regular breast self-examinations monthly after 20 years of age.
- A physician should examine clients from 20 years of age to 40 years of age every 3 years and clients older than 40 years of age annually.
- Women with a family history of breast cancer should be examined annually by a physician.
- Always perform examinations the last day of the menstrual period or the same day each month if the client has reached menopause.
- A diagnostic mammogram (x-ray examination of the breast) should be performed every 1 to 2 years for women aged 40 to 50 years; every year for women older than 50 years of age; and every year for women 40 years of age or older with a family history of breast cancer.
- Discuss signs and symptoms of breast cancer.

Abdomen

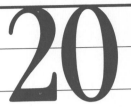

Anatomy and Physiology

Within the abdominal cavity are located various organs of numerous body systems (Fig. 42). The stomach, located in the left upper abdominal quadrant under the costal margin, is a hollow organ that digests and stores food before it passes through the intestines. The small and large intestines, which function to absorb water and nutrients, secrete substances to promote digestion and passage of contents, and eliminate wastes, course throughout the abdominal cavity.

The kidneys are located deep in both upper quadrants of the abdomen. These organs selectively filter, reabsorb, and secrete water and electrolytes delivered by means of the circulatory system to maintain fluid and electrolyte balance and eliminate wastes.

The liver, one of the most important organs of the body, is located in the right upper quadrant just above the costal margin. Its functions include the formation of serum protein; production of bile; metabolism of fat, carbohydrate, and protein; detoxification of foreign substances; and metabolism of bilirubin.

The bladder is a hollow, distensible organ that collects and eliminates urine formed by the kidneys. Normally it lies below the symphysis pubis, but once it becomes distended it can become palpable just above the pubic bone.

Tissues and bones outside the abdominal cavity (for example, the spine and muscles) protect vital organs. These structures may be involved when clients have abdominal pain.

Rationale

The abdominal examination primarily includes an assessment of structures of the lower gastrointestinal (GI) tract in addition to the liver, stomach, kidneys, and bladder. Disturbances in a person's bowel elimination pattern can often be detected during an

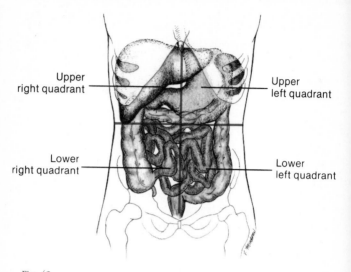

Fig. 42
Position of underlying abdominal organs in relation to anatomic landmarks.
(From Potter PA and Perry AG: Fundamentals of nursing: concepts, process, and practice, ed 2, St Louis, 1989, The CV Mosby Co.)

abdominal assessment. Since many factors influence bowel function, for example, dietary changes, medications, stress, or surgery, the nurse can use assessment findings in caring for a variety of health problems. The nurse's assessment of the abdomen determines the presence or absence of masses, tenderness, organ enlargement, and peristaltic activity.

When assessing the abdomen the nurse uses a system of landmarks to map out the abdominal region. The nurse imagines the abdomen as divided into four equal quadrants, with the xiphoid process (tip of sternum) marking the upper boundary and the symphysis pubis delineating the lowermost boundary. Two imaginary lines cross at the umbilicus to form the quadrants. Assessment findings are recorded in relation to the quadrants. For example, pain may be noted in the lower left quadrant (LLQ).

Abdominal Assessment
Special Equipment

The following equipment is used in assessing the abdomen:

Stethoscope

Adequate lighting

Small ruler

Marking pencil

Small pillow

Client Preparation

- To help the client relax, offer an opportunity to void before beginning the examination.
- The room should be warm and the client's upper chest and legs should be draped.
- Expose the abdomen from just above the xiphoid process to the symphysis pubis.
- Make sure lighting is good.
- The client lies supine with arms down at the side or folded across the chest. A small pillow may be placed under the head or knees.
- Keep your hands and the stethoscope warm to help the client relax.

History

- If the client has abdominal or lower back pain, assess the character of pain in detail, including location, quality, onset, frequency, aggravating factors, severity, and precipitating factors such as meal ingestion.
- Ask about the client's normal bowel habits and stool character. Ask whether the client uses laxatives frequently.
- Note the client's movement and position, such as lying with the knees drawn up or moving restlessly to find a comfortable position; this can reveal the nature and source of pain.
- Ask whether the client has had abdominal surgery, trauma, or gastrointestinal (GI) diagnostic tests.
- Ask whether the client has had a recent weight change, intolerance to diet, for example, nausea, vomiting, cramping, or a change in appetite.
- Note any belching, difficulty in swallowing, flatulence, bloody emesis (hematemesis), or black or tarry stools (melena).
- Ask whether the client takes medications such as aspirin or steroids that may affect GI integrity.

Assessment Techniques

The order of an abdominal assessment differs from other body system reviews. Begin with inspection, then follow with auscultation. Auscultate before palpation or percussion to ensure accurate assessment of bowel sounds.

Assessment	Normal Findings
Stand at client's right side and inspect from above the abdomen to detect abnormal shadows and movement.	
Bend down and inspect the abdomen from a lower position to detect abnormal protuberances.	Abdomen's shape is symmetric.
Inspect skin over abdomen for scars, venous patterns, lesions, and stretch marks (striae).	Venous patterns are normally faint except in thin clients. Striae result from stretching tissue by obesity or pregnancy.
Inspect shape and symmetry of the abdomen and note any masses or distention.	A flat abdomen forms a horizontal plane from the xiphoid process to the symphysis pubis. A round abdomen is convex. A concave abdomen seems to sink into the muscular wall.
If the abdomen seems distended, ask the client to roll onto side and inspect for bulging flank; ask client whether abdomen feels unusually tight.	Temporary distention can be caused by a heavy meal. Do not confuse distention with obesity, marked by rolls of adipose tissue along the flanks and no client report of tightness.
If abdominal distention is expected, measure abdomen's girth by placing a tape measure around abdomen at umbilicus. Consecutive measurements will show any change.	

Assessment	Normal Findings
Inspect abdomen for normal respiratory movement.	Males breathe more abdominally than costally. Females breathe more costally.
Inspect umbilicus for position, shape, color, and any discharge or protruding mass.	The umbilicus is normally a flat or concave hemisphere, positioned midway between the xiphoid and symphysis pubis. Color is same as surrounding skin. There is normally no discharge from the umbilicus.
Observe abdominal contour while asking client to take a deep breath.	No bulges appear.
Note presence of peristaltic movement or aortic pulsation.	Visible in very thin clients, otherwise no movement is present.
Place the warmed diaphragm of the stethoscope over each of the four quadrants. Ask the client not to speak. Listen for bowel sounds. It may take 3 to 5 minutes before the examiner decides bowel sounds are absent.	Bowel sounds are high pitched and irregular. Gurgling or bubbling sounds in each quadrant are normally caused by air and fluid moving through the intestines.
It normally takes 5 to 20 seconds to hear a bowel sound, but it can take up to 1 minute.	Bowel sounds normally last about ½ second each. Series of bowel sounds last several seconds.
Record the client's bowel sounds as normal or audible, absent, hyperactive, or hypoactive.	
Using the stethoscope bell, the examiner should auscultate the thoracic aorta for bruits.	Normally there are no vascular sounds over the aorta or renal artery.

Assessment	Normal Findings
	Nurse Alert
Place the stethoscope over each upper quadrant anteriorly to hear for renal artery bruits.	If bruits are heard do not palpate the abdomen. Injury to an underlying aneurysm may result.
Percuss over all four quadrants and note percussion tones.	Hollow organs such as the stomach, intestine, bladder, and aorta are tympanic. A dull tone can be heard over the liver, spleen, pancreas, kidneys, and a distended bladder.
Use percussion to locate borders of underlying organs.	

Liver

Assessment	Normal Findings
Stand on client's right side and begin to percuss at the right midclavicular line just below the umbilicus. Slowly percuss upward.	Note changes from tympanic to dull once you percuss the liver's lower border. Usually the border is at the right costal margin.
To locate the upper border, percuss downward from the clavicle at the intercostal space. Then note changes from resonant to dull.	The liver's upper border is usually at the fifth, sixth, or seventh intercostal space. Distance between upper and lower border is 6 to 12 cm (2½ to 5 inches).

Stomach

Assessment	Normal Findings
Percuss over the lower left anterior rib cage.	The stomach's air bubble is tympanic.

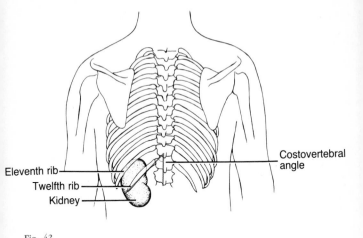

Fig. 43
Kidneys normally lie behind lower ribs at a point even with costovertebral angle.
(From Potter PA and Perry AG: Fundamentals of nursing: concepts, process, and practice, ed 2, St Louis, 1989, The CV Mosby Co.)

Kidney

Assessment	Normal Findings
Ask the client to sit or stand. Percuss the costovertebral angle at the scapular line (Fig. 43). Palpate the abdomen lightly over each of the four quadrants.	Percussion is painless; the client feels only a slight sensation of pressure.
Depressing the skin approximately ½ inch (1.2 cm), palpate to detect areas of tenderness and any abnormal distention or mass. During palpation watch client's face for any signs of discomfort.	Abdomen is normally soft and nontender without masses. A distended bladder may be felt just below the umbilicus.

Assessment	Normal Findings
Avoid any quick jabs during palpation.	
Use deep palpation (experienced nurses only), depressing the skin 1 to 3 inches (2.5 to 7.5 cm), to palpate deep masses—never use deep palpation over tender organs or a surgical incision.	No masses are felt.
Note the characteristics of any deep mass, including size, location, shape, consistency, tenderness, and mobility.	
If tenderness is found, test for rebound tenderness: press deeply and then release quickly to detect whether pain is elicited by releasing pressure.	
Attempt to palpate the liver's edge as follows: standing at the client's right side, place your left hand under the client's right posterior thorax at the 11th and 12th ribs. Apply upward pressure.	The liver is usually difficult to palpate in a normal adult. On palpation, the liver is nontender and smooth and has a regular contour with a sharp edge.
Place the fingers of the right hand pointing toward the right costal margin and placed below the liver's lower border. Press gently in and up with the right hand. Ask the client to inhale and try to feel the liver's edge as it descends.	Liver is nontender and has a firm, regular, sharp edge.

Assessment	Normal Findings
To palpate for aortic pulsation, use the thumb and forefinger of one hand. Palpate slowly but deeply into the upper abdomen just left of the midline. If it is suspected that a client has ascites, an accumulation of serous fluid in the peritoneal cavity, place the palmar surface of the fingers and hand firmly on one side of abdomen. Use the other hand to tap the opposite abdominal wall. Note whether tapping causes a fluid wave to be felt by the flattened hand.	Normal pulsation is transmitted.

Deviations from Normal

Abdominal scars may indicate past trauma or surgery that changed underlying organ anatomy.

Record any skin lesion findings as described in Chapter 10. Asymmetry of the abdomen or one-sided masses may indicate an underlying pathologic condition.

Hernias can cause an upward protrusion of the umbilicus.

Underlying masses can displace the umbilicus.

Abdominal distention may be caused by intestinal gas, tumor, or fluid in the abdominal cavity.

Distention is marked by tightly stretched skin.

Fluid distention causes the dependent flank to bulge when client rolls on side; gas distention does not.

Diminished respiratory movement of the abdomen may be caused by guarding against pain.

Absent bowel sounds indicate a cessation of gastric motility.

Hyperactive bowel sounds (borborygmi) indicate increased gastric motility, caused by bowel inflammation, excessive laxative use, and reactions to certain foods or hunger.

Aortic bruits may indicate the narrowing of the aorta or an aneurysm.

An enlarged liver may indicate liver disease.

A smooth, nontender, enlarged liver is a sign of cirrhosis.

Sharp pain or tenderness on percussion of the kidneys indicates inflammation.

Guarding may be elicited by palpation of any tender area.

Rebound tenderness may indicate inflammation of the abdominal cavity (peritonitis).

Enlargement of the aorta from an aneurysm causes the pulsation to expand laterally.

With ascites, a fluid wave is palpated.

Nursing Diagnosis

Assessment data may reveal the following diagnoses:

- Constipation related to a change in eating habits or medication.
- Pain related to abdominal inflammation.
- Altered nutrition: less or more than body requirements related to dietary habits.
- Knowledge deficit regarding the use of laxatives related to misinformation.

Pediatric Considerations

- Distraction is important to help children relax when assessing them. Involve the child's parents.
- A child may confuse the pressure of palpation with pain. Children are also often ticklish.
- Visible peristaltic waves warrant careful evaluation and can indicate intestinal obstruction.
- Organs palpable in children include the bladder, cecum, and sigmoid colon.

Gerontologic Considerations

- Normally elderly clients have reduced gastrointestinal motility, and constipation is a common problem.

Client Teaching

- Explain factors that promote normal bowel elimination, such as diet, regular exercise, and fluid intake.
- Caution the client about the dangers of excessive use of laxatives or enemas.
- If the client has chronic pain, explain measures for pain relief.

Female and Male Genitalia

21

Female Genitalia

Assessment of the female genitalia consists of examination of external genitalia and speculum examination of internal genitalia described separately in the following sections.

Anatomy and Physiology

The female genitalia consist of external and internal sex organs. The external sex organs, referred to collectively as the vulva, include the mons veneris, labia majora, labia minora, clitoris, and vaginal opening (Fig. 44). The internal sex organs include the vagina, uterus, fallopian tubes, and ovaries.

Vulva

The mons veneris is a layer of fatty tissue that covers the pubic bone and is covered by pubic hair in the postpubescent female. The two labia majora are fatty folds of skin whose outer surfaces are covered with pubic hair and whose inner surfaces are smooth and hairless. The labia majora extend down from the mons veneris and form the outer boundaries of the vulva. They have sensory receptors that are sensitive to touch, pressure, pain, and temperature. The two labia minora, which are just inside the labia majora, are thin folds of pigmented skin that extend upward to form the clitoral hood. These inner folds possess many blood vessels and have many sensory nerve endings.

Clitoris

When the clitoral hood is pulled back, the glans of the clitoris is revealed. It looks like a smooth, shiny pea. The clitoris has many nerve endings and is very sensitive to touch, pressure, and temperature.

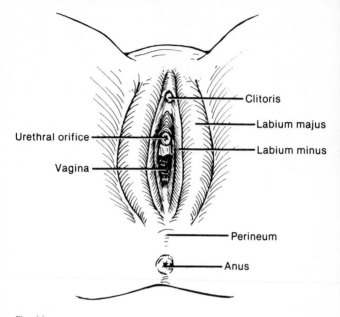

Fig. 44
External female sex organs.
(From Potter PA and Perry AG: Fundamentals of nursing: concepts, process, and practice, ed 2, St Louis, The CV Mosby Co.)

Introitus

The vaginal opening, or introitus, is between the urethra and the anus. The hymen is a membranous fold of tissue that partially covers the introitus. It has no known function. It usually remains intact until the first intercourse.

The Bartholin's glands are two small ducts that open on the inner surface of the labia minora next to the vaginal opening. The Bartholin's glands secrete a small amount of lubricating fluid.

Vagina

The vagina is a thin-walled, muscular organ that tilts upward at a 45-degree angle toward the small of the back. The walls of the vagina consist of a thin outer serosa; a middle layer of smooth, involuntary muscle that is continuous with the muscle of the uterus; and an inner layer of moist mucous membrane called mucosa. The vagina serves as a passageway for menstrual flow and childbirth.

Uterus

The uterus is a thick-walled muscular organ located between the urinary bladder and rectum. It is about 3 inches (7.5 cm) long and looks like a small pear turned upside down. The fallopian tubes enter the uterus on either side near the top. The wide upper part of the uterus is known as the body. The bottom part, called the cervix, protrudes into the vagina. The inner lining of the cervix contains many glands that secrete varying amounts of mucus that plug the opening to the uterus.

Fallopian tubes

The two fallopian tubes begin at the uterus and end in long fingerlike fimbriae near the ovaries. The chief function of the fallopian tubes is as a conduit for the passage of both egg and sperm so that fertilization can take place.

Ovaries

The two walnut-sized ovaries, one on each side of the uterus, have two functions. They produce eggs that are released into the fallopian tubes, and they secrete female hormones, including small amounts of androgen, directly into the bloodstream.

Rationale

Examination of the genitalia should be a part of all preventive health care examinations because women have a high incidence of uterine and vaginal cancer. All women older than 20 years of age should have yearly examinations. Assessment of the genitalia also serves to screen for incidence of sexually transmitted disease. The external genitalia may be assessed during a separate examination, routine hygiene measures, or the insertion of a urinary catheter.

Genitalia Assessment
Special equipment

Examination table with stirrups
Vaginal speculum of correct size
Adjustable light source

Sink
Lubricant
Clean disposable gloves
Glass microscope slides
Sponge forceps or swabs
Wood spatulas
Specimen bottle with fixative

Client preparation

- Have the client empty her bladder before the examination so that a specimen may be obtained.

Make sure the client is emotionally prepared because genital examination is often viewed with fear or apprehension. Because the client may be embarrassed by the lithotomy position, use a calm, reassuring, and attentive approach, position and drape the client carefully, explain each part of the examination in advance, and avoid any delays or interruptions during assessment.

Help the client into a lithotomy position, in bed or on the examining table for an external genitalia assessment only. Use the stirrups if the speculum examination is to be performed. If the client has pain or deformity of the joints, only one leg may be abducted or another nurse can assist by separating the client's thighs. Offer a pillow for the client's head. Drape the client such that one corner of the drape covers the perineal area until the examination begins.

A male examiner should have a female assistant in attendance, and a female examiner should also be accompanied if the client is particularly anxious or emotionally unstable.

History

- Has the client had previous illness or surgery involving reproductive organs, including sexually transmitted diseases?
- Review menstrual history, including age at menarche, frequency and duration of menstrual cycle, character of flow, presence of pain, and dates of last two menstrual periods.
- Ask the client to describe obstetric history, that is, have her describe each pregnancy and her history of abortions and miscarriages.
- Have the client describe current and past contraceptive practices.
- Does the client have symptoms of genitourinary problems such

as dysuria, frequency, urgency, nocturia, hematuria, incontinence, or stress incontinence?
- Assess client's sexual history.
- Has client noted any vaginal discharge, painful or swollen perianal tissues, or lesions of the genitalia?

Assessment techniques
External genitalia

Assessment	Normal Findings
Adjust light so that the perineal area is well illuminated.	The perineal skin is slightly darker than other skin.
Put gloves on both hands.	In an adult, hair growth forms a triangle over the perineum and along the medial surface of the thighs.
Do not touch the perineal area without warning the client, or touch one thigh first and advance to the perineum.	Mucous membranes appear dark pink and moist.
Inspect quantity and distribution of hair growth.	The labia majora are usually plump and well formed in adult women.
Inspect the appearance of the labia majora.	After menopause, the labia majora become thinner.
	After childbirth, the labia majora are separated and the labia minora are more prominent.
	The labia become atrophied with advancing age.
Gently retract tissues of labia majora outward to inspect the clitoris, labia minora, urethral orifice, hymen, and vaginal orifice.	The labia minora are normally thinner than the labia majora, and one side may be larger.
Inspect the clitoris and labia minora for size and shape.	The size of the clitoris is variable, but the clitoris normally does not exceed 0.5 cm in diameter.
Observe urethral orifice carefully for color and position.	The urethral meatus is anterior to the vaginal orifice and is pink.

Assessment	Normal Findings
If inflammation is suspected, check for urethral discharge by placing index finger inside vaginal orifice and gently milking the urethra from inside outward.	In virgins, the labia minora lie together. After childbirth or intercourse, the labia tend to gape or fall to the side.
If urethral drainage is present, change to a clean pair of gloves.	Urethral orifice is normally intact without inflammation.
Note the condition of the hymen.	
Inspect posterior end of vaginal introitus for inflammation or edema.	In women who have had several children, the opening to the vagina canal may extend upward obstructing the view of the urethra.
	In virgins the hymen may restrict the opening of the vagina.
	Only remnants of the hymen remain after sexual intercourse.
Attempt to palpate the Bartholin's glands one side at a time with thumb and index finger between labia majora and introitus.	The Bartholin's glands normally cannot be palpated.
Ask the client to strain downward as if voiding to assess for loss of support of the vaginal outlet.	During straining there should be no bulging of tissue through the vaginal orifice.
If rectal examination is to be included, proceed with this assessment at this time (see Chapter 22).	

Deviations from Normal	Nurse Alert
Inflammation, edema, lesions, or lacerations of the labia majora are abnormal findings.	

Deviations from Normal	Nurse Alert
Bright red color of the clitoris indicates inflammation.	
Syphilitic lesions or chancres may appear as small open ulcers draining serous material.	
Dry, scaly, nodular lesions in elderly clients may be malignant changes.	
Drainage manually expressed from the urethra indicates inflammation and infection.	
Inflammation and edema near the posterior end of the introitus may indicate infection of the Bartholin's glands.	
Bulging of the vaginal walls that blocks the introitus when the client strains indicates lack of support of the vaginal outlet.	The appearance of a large tissue mass in the vaginal opening when the client strains should be reported immediately. This may indicate prolapse of uterus or bladder.

Speculum examination

Speculum examination requires considerable practice and should not be performed by inexperienced persons without supervision.

Rationale

The speculum examination is performed to assess the internal genitalia for cancerous lesions and other abnormalities and to collect specimens for a Pap smear to test for cervical and vaginal cancer. Women who are older than 20 years of age and have no symptoms of disease and sexually active women younger than 20 years of age should have annual Pap smears until two tests are negative and thereafter every 3 years until 65 years of age. Women at risk for cervical cancer should have annual checkups. Risk factors include family history of disease, exposure to herpesvirus type 2, first coitus at an early age, and multiple sexual partners.

Assessment	Normal Findings

Select the proper size speculum and warm it in running water.

Use water as the lubricant because commercial lubricants can interfere with Pap smear studies.

Apply a pair of disposable gloves.

Adjust light source over your shoulder to the examination site.

Explain to the client what you are doing during the examination.

If client has never had a speculum examination, first insert two fingers of non-dominant hand into vagina to explore for abnormalities.

With the two fingers press down on the perineal body just inside the introitus.

With speculum blades closed, holding speculum in dominant hand, insert speculum obliquely (rotated 50 degrees counterclockwise from vertical) past your fingers downward at a 45-degree angle toward the examination table (Fig. 45).

Take care to avoid pulling pubic hair or pinching the labia.

When the blades are inside the introitus, rotate the speculum so that the blades are horizontal.

Client may feel some discomfort as vaginal opening is stretched.

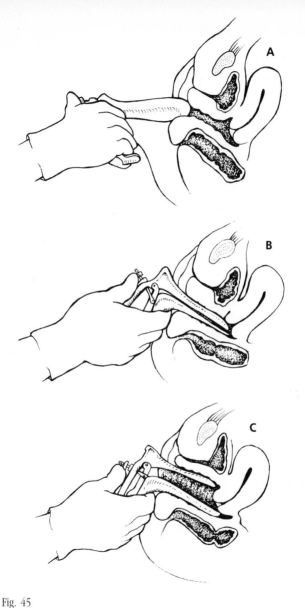

Fig. 45

Insertion of vaginal speculum. **A,** Speculum introduced at oblique angle. **B,** Speculum inserted downward at 45° angle to table. **C,** Blades are opened after full insertion.

(From Potter PA and Perry AG: Fundamentals of nursing: concepts, process, and practice, ed 2, St Louis, 1989, The CV Mosby Co.)

Assessment	Normal Findings
Open the blades slowly to view the cervix and lock the blades in open position.	The cervix is normally a glistening pink smooth, round, depressed area with a diameter of about 1 inch (2.5 to 3 cm) in a young woman, smaller in an elderly female.
Inspect cervix for color, contour, position, size, and symmetry. Inspect opening (os) for size and presence of any abnormalities.	
Describe any irregularities or lesions as being in a 12 o'clock position, 6 o'clock position, and so forth around the cervix.	The cervix becomes pale after menopause and cyanotic during pregnancy.
Assess any discharge for color, odor, quantity, and consistency.	The os is usually small and closed in women who have not had children or larger and slightly curved following childbirth. In multiparous women the cervical os may have gaps.
Collect Pap smear specimens from three sites:	
Endocervical area: Use cotton swab or cotton-tipped applicator and gently swab through cervical os, rotating 360 degrees.	
Outer cervix: Use a wooden Ayre spatula, placing the tip of the longer arm in cervical os, then rotating spatula and scraping the outer surface of the cervix.	
Vaginal pool: Place handle of spatula into vagina and rotate against vaginal floor.	
With all three specimens, apply cells and secretions to glass microscope slides, apply fixative solution, and label with the client's name and the specimen source.	Normal results on the Pap smear are negative.
Inspect the vaginal walls while withdrawing the speculum with the set screw loose but the blades held open.	

Assessment	Normal Findings
Inspect the vaginal wall's color, texture, and support; record any discharge or lesions.	The vaginal walls are normally pink throughout and free of discharge and lesions.
Close speculum blades gradually during removal to prevent excessive stretching and pinching.	
Proceed to rectal examination (see Chapter 22) or complete this assessment by cleansing the perineum and anal area to remove any moisture or drainage.	

Deviations from Normal

Cervical discharge, lacerations, ulcerations, or lesions are abnormal.

Chronic cervical infections cause thick, malodorous discharges.

A thick, white, patchy, curdlike substance clinging to vaginal walls indicates a yeast infection.

Positive Pap smear results indicate the presence of abnormal cells and may require further diagnostic testing.

Nursing diagnosis

Assessment data may reveal the following diagnoses:

- Stress or urge incontinence related to neuromuscular impairment.
- Sexual dysfunction related to altered body structure.
- Knowledge deficit regarding birth control methods, effects of menopause, and the need for pelvic examinations related to inexperience.

Gerontologic considerations

Vaginal epithelium is thinner, drier, and less vascular, and the cervix and uterus become smaller.

Client teaching

- Instruct the client about recommended frequency of Pap smears and gynecologic examinations.
- Counsel clients with sexually transmitted diseases about diag-

nosis and treatment. Teach preventive measures, for example, male partners' use of condoms, restricting the number of sexual partners, avoiding sex with persons who have several other partners, and perineal hygiene measures.

- Tell clients with sexually transmitted diseases that they must inform sexual partners of the need for an examination.
- Reinforce the importance of perineal hygiene.
- Explore with clients alternate sources of sexual satisfaction.
- Discuss optional forms of birth control.

Male Genitalia

Examination of the male genitalia includes assessing the integrity of external genitalia and the inguinal ring and canal.

Anatomy and Physiology

The external male genitalia are the penis and scrotum. The male internal sex organs include the testicles, which produce hormones and sperm; the epididymis and vas deferens, a system of ducts that transport sperm; and the prostate gland, seminal vesicles, and Cowper's glands, whose secretions become part of the ejaculated semen (Fig. 46).

Penis

The penis consists of the shaft, which is composed primarily of erectile tissue, and the glans, which has both erectile and sensory tissue. The penile shaft comprises three parallel tubes: two corpora cavernosa, which lie side by side, and beneath them a single corpus spongiosum, which surrounds the urethra.

The anterior end of the corpus spongiosum fits over the corpora cavernosa and is called the glans. The glans resembles an acorn. The area where the glans arises abruptly from the shaft is called the corona, meaning crown. If the male is uncircumcised, the skin of the shaft continues forward and forms a loose-fitting hood over the glans. This hood is called the foreskin or prepuce. On the undersurface the glans is attached to the prepuce by a thin fold of skin called the frenulum.

Scrotum

The scrotum is a thin, loose sac of skin that protects the two testicles. It is located at the base of the penis. The scrotum is di-

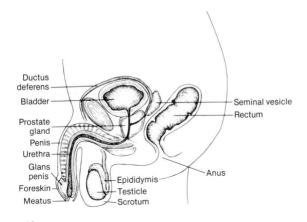

Fig. 46

Male sex organs.

(From Potter PA and Perry AG: Fundamentals of nursing: concepts, process, and practice, ed 2, St Louis, 1989, The CV Mosby Co.)

vided into two compartments, each containing a testis, epididymis, and part of the vas deferens. The testis, epididymis, and parts of the vas deferens that are in the scrotum are considered internal organs even though they are outside the body cavity.

Internal sex organs

The left testicle usually hangs lower than the right testicle. The testicles have two main functions: to produce sperm and to produce hormones.

The sperm drain into the epididymis, a duct that lies just outside the testicle. The vas deferens is a long tube from each testicle that goes up and out of the scrotum. It curves around the urinary bladder and then turns downward and opens into an enlargement 4 inches (10 cm) long called the ampulla. The ampulla is a reservoir for the sperm before they are discharged into the ejaculatory duct, which carries them through the prostate into the posterior urethra. The urethra goes from the bladder to the penis tip and carries urine or semen.

The prostate is about the size of a chestnut and is located beneath the bladder. The ejaculatory ducts and a portion of the urethra pass through it.

Genitalia Assessment
Rationale

Because of the high incidence of sexually transmitted disease in adolescents and young adults, the genitalia should be assessed routinely during health maintenance examinations.

Special equipment

Disposable gloves

Client preparation

- Ask client whether he needs to empty his bladder.
- Make sure the room is warm.
- Have the client lie supine with the chest, abdomen, and lower legs draped. The client may also stand during the examination.
- Because the client may feel anxious during the examination, particularly with a female nurse, help him relax and explain each step of the examination.

History

- Assess normal urinary pattern, including frequency of voiding; history of nocturia; character and volume of urine; daily fluid intake; symptoms of burning, urgency, and frequency; difficulty starting stream; and hematuria.
- Assess client's sexual history.
- Determine whether the client has had previous surgery or illness involving urinary or reproductive organs.
- Has client noted penile pain or swelling, lesions of genitalia, or urethral discharge?

Assessment techniques

Assessment	Normal Findings
Apply disposable gloves	
Assess the sexual maturity of the client; note size and shape of penis, size, color, and texture of scrotal skin, and character and distribution of pubic hair.	First increase in size of testes occurs at 9.5 years of age to 13.5 years of age. During preadolescence no pubic hair.

Assessment	Normal Findings
	By end of puberty testes and penis enlarge to adult size and shape, scrotal skin darkens and becomes wrinkled.
Inspect the skin covering the genitalia for lice, rashes, excoriations, or lesions.	Skin clear without lesions.
Manipulate the genitalia gently to avoid discomfort.	Penile erection may occur during examination with manipulation of penile structures.
Inspect the structures constituting the penis.	
In uncircumcised males, retract the foreskin to inspect the glans and urethral meatus for discharge, lesions, edema, and inflammation. Inspect the glans around its entire circumference for signs of lesions.	The meatus is normally positioned at the tip of the glans. The glans is smooth and pink. A small amount of thick white secretion is normal between the glans and foreskin.
Gentle compression of the glans between the thumb and index finger opens the urethral meatus to inspect for discharge, lesions, and edema.	No discharge present.
Palpate any lesion gently to note tenderness, size, consistency, and shape. Pull retracted foreskin down to its original position.	
Inspect the shaft of the penis, not overlooking its undersurface, for any lesions, scars, or areas of edema.	A client who has lain in bed for a prolonged time may develop dependent edema in the penile shaft.

Assessment	Normal Findings
Gently palpate the shaft between thumb and first two fingers to note any localized areas of hardness.	
Be particularly gentle when touching the scrotum.	
Inspect the scrotum's size, shape, and symmetry, and observe for lesions or edema.	The left testis may normally be lower than the right.
Gently lift scrotum to view posterior surface.	The skin of the scrotum is normally loose.
	The scrotum normally contracts in cold temperatures and relaxes in warm temperatures.
Gently palpate the testes and epididymis between thumb and first two fingers and note size, shape, and consistency; ask client whether palpation reveals any unusual tenderness.	The testes are normally oval shaped and approximately ½ to 1 inch (1 to 2 cm) in diameter.
	The testes feel smooth, firm, and the epididymides feel resilient.
Continue to palpate the vas deferens separately as it forms the spermatic cord toward the inguinal ring.	Without nodules or swelling.
Ask client to stand for assessment of the inguinal ring and canal.	
During inspection, ask the client to bear down.	Abdominal muscles tighten and scrotum lowers as client bears down.
Inspect both inguinal areas for signs of obvious bulging caused by hernia through inguinal ring or canal.	

Assessment	Normal Findings
Palpate the inguinal ring and canal to be sure a hernia is not present: Begin by gently invaginating the scrotal skin on the right side, starting at a point low on the scrotum. Follow the spermatic cord up to the inguinal ring. Do not force finger into inguinal canal.	
When the finger reaches the farthest point along the canal, ask client to cough and strain down. Repeat on left side.	As client strains, no bulging pressure will be felt against fingertips; a tightening around the finger is normal.
Palpate the prostate gland during rectal examination (see Chapter 22).	

Deviations from Normal

In some congenital conditions the meatus is displaced along the penile shaft.

The area between foreskin and glans is a common site for venereal lesions.

Tight scrotal skin may indicate edema.

An abnormally large scrotal sac may indicate inguinal hernia, hydrocele, or inflammation of internal structures.

A small, hard lump about the size of a pea, on the front side of the testicle is the most common symptom of testicular cancer.

If the client has a hernia, it will protrude against the finger at the inguinal canal on coughing.

If any signs of venereal disease or other lesions are found, the client should be referred to his physician.

Nursing diagnosis

Assessment data may reveal the following nursing diagnoses:
- Pain related to inflammatory lesions.
- Knowledge deficit regarding testicular self-examination related to inexperience.
- Altered patterns of urinary elimination related to infection.
- Sexual dysfunction related to lack of knowledge.

Pediatric considerations

With children and presexual female adolescents, assessment is only of external genitalia.

Uncircumcised infants (2 to 3 months of age) should not have foreskin retracted because of risk of tearing membrane.

Undescended testes are common in premature infants.

With adolescents, genital examination may be left until last because adolescents are more likely to be embarrassed. The examiner should proceed calmly as with all other segments of the examination.

Gerontologic considerations

The size and firmness of the testes generally decrease with age.

Client teaching

If the client expresses interest or concern about sexually transmitted disease, contraceptive techniques, physiologic functioning, and other matters of human sexuality, the nurse may choose to provide information following the examination.

Rectum

22

For both male and female clients, assessment of the rectum can generally best be performed immediately following assessment of the genitalia. For males, rectal assessment includes assessment of the prostate gland.

Anatomy and Physiology

The rectum is the terminal portion of the lower gastrointestinal tract. Basically, it is a hollow tube, 4 to 6 inches (10 to 15 cm) in length containing folds of mucus-lined tissue. Its role is to function in the elimination of solid wastes through the defecation reflex. The defecation reflex is under both involuntary and voluntary control.

Rationale

The primary purpose of the rectal examination is for determining the presence of masses or irregularities of the rectal walls. The integrity of the external anal sphincter can also be assessed. In males the rectal examination provides access to assess the condition of the prostate gland. Prostatic cancer is the second most common form of cancer among men.

Rectal Assessment
Special Equipment

Disposable gloves
Lubricant

Client Preparation

- The examination can be uncomfortable and embarrassing; use a calm, gentle approach.
- The female client is assessed in the lithotomy position if rectal assessment follows vaginal examination. Otherwise the female should assume a side-lying, or Sims', position.

- The male client is asked to bend forward with hips flexed and upper body resting across the examination table.
- Nonambulatory male clients may be assessed in the Sims' position.

History

- Has client experienced bleeding from the rectum, black or tarry stools (melena), rectal pain, or change in bowel habits (constipation or diarrhea)?
- Determine whether the client has personal or family history of colorectal cancer, polyps, or inflammatory bowel disease.
- Assess dietary habits for high fat intake or deficient fiber content that may be linked to bowel cancer.
- Has the client ever undergone screening for colorectal cancer?
- Assess medication history for use of laxatives or cathartics, codeine, or iron preparations.

Assessment Techniques

Assessment	Normal Findings
Apply disposable gloves and with nondominant hand retract buttocks to inspect the perianal area for lumps, hemorrhoids, ulcers, inflammation, rashes, or excoriations.	Anal tissues are moist and hairless. Anus is held closed by the voluntary sphincter. Perianal tissue is intact and more pigmented and coarser than skin overlying buttocks.
Ask client to bear down (note presence of internal hemorrhoids or fissures).	No protrusion of tissue. **Nurse Alert** Some institutions do not permit nurses to perform digital examinations.
Apply lubricant to gloved index finger of nondominant hand.	
Insert finger into anal canal by asking client to bear down as though having a bowel movement. As the anal sphincter relaxes, insert fingertip gently into the anal canal directed toward the umbilicus.	While assessor's finger is inserted, client may have sensation of need to have a bowel movement.

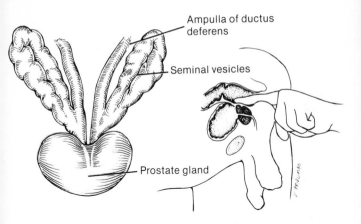

Fig. 47
Palpation of prostate gland during rectal examination.

Assessment	Normal Findings
Note the tone of the anal sphincter.	Muscles close snugly around finger.
Carefully palpate each side of the rectal wall and note any nodules, lesions, hemorrhoids, or irregularities. Ask client whether tenderness is felt. When finger is fully advanced, ask client to bear down to detect any high lesions.	Wall of rectum is usually smooth. Stool is commonly found in the rectum.
Test sphincter tone by asking client to tighten muscles around finger.	Sphincter normally closes around finger.
In male clients turn the index finger to palpate the anterior rectal wall. Palpate prostate gland to determine size, shape, firmness, tenderness, or lesions (Fig. 47).	Male prostate is round and heart shaped, 1 to 1.5 inches (2.5 to 4 cm) in diameter, divided into two lobes by a small groove, firm, and nontender.

Assessment	Normal Findings

Gently withdraw finger.

Stool on gloved finger can be guaiac tested for occult blood.

Complete the examination by cleansing the anal and perineal area.

Deviations from Normal

Tenderness, lesions, nodules, hemorrhoids, or other irregularities in anal canal.

External hemorrhoids lie around anal orifice.

Lesions high in anal canal may descend against examiner's finger when the client bears down.

Abnormal findings in male prostate include boggy consistency, tenderness, hardness, or nodules.

Nursing Diagnosis

Assessment data may reveal the following nursing diagnoses:
- Knowledge deficit regarding risks for colorectal cancer related to inexperience.
- Pain related to hemorrhoid inflammation.
- Constipation related to rectal pain.
- Anxiety related to the threat of cancer diagnosis.

Pediatric Considerations

In the neonate, passage of meconium stool within the first 48 hours of life indicates anal patency.

Parents should be assured that toilet training is individualized for children and cannot begin until the child has mature neurologic and muscular development.

Gerontologic Considerations

Most older men have some degree of prostatic enlargement and require biannual examination and close follow-up to manage the recurrent urinary tract infections and to ensure that carcinoma does not exist.

Client Teaching

- Discuss the American Cancer Society's guidelines for early detection of colorectal cancer, including digital rectal examina-

tions performed yearly after 40 years of age; stool blood slide
tests (guaiac test) performed yearly after 50 years of age; proctosigmoidoscopy, involving visual inspection of the rectum and
lower colon with a hollow, lighted tube. Proctosigmoidoscopy
is performed by a physician every 3 to 5 years after 50 years of
age and after two annual examinations with negative results.

- Discuss diet plan to reduce fat and increase fiber content.
- Warn client about problems caused by overuse of laxatives, cathartics, codeine, and enemas.

Musculoskeletal System

23

Musculoskeletal assessment can be conducted as a separate examination or integrated appropriately with other parts of the total physical examination. The nurse can also integrate this assessment with other nursing care as the client moves about or practices range of motion exercises.

Musculoskeletal assessment consists of general inspection and assessment of range of joint motion, muscle tone, and muscle strength, described separately in the following sections.

Anatomy and Physiology

An understanding of the anatomy and physiology of all structures of the musculoskeletal system goes beyond the scope of this text. The primary structures are the bones, muscles, cartilage, ligaments, tendons, and joints. Each works in synchrony to provide flexible, fluid movement of body parts. The bones also protect underlying vital organs and support the body's skeletal framework.

Rationale

The integrity of the musculoskeletal system is vital for persons to move about freely and care for themselves. Disorders of the musculoskeletal system can range from alterations causing minor discomfort, such as sprained ligaments, to life-threatening conditions, such as muscular dystrophy. The nurse's examination includes assessment of the bones, supportive tissues, such as cartilage, tendons, and fasciae, muscles, and joints. The nurse gives particular attention to areas of limited or absent movement to determine the level and extent of a client's disability. The client may exhibit problems resulting from disease of bones or joints, trauma, or disorders of the nerves that innervate the musculoskeletal system.

Musculoskeletal Assessment
Special Equipment

The following equipment is needed when assessing the musculoskeletal system:

Goniometer

Tape measure

Client Preparation

- Depending on the muscle groups assessed, the client sits, lies supine, or stands.
- Be sure the client's muscles and joints are exposed and free to move.

History

- Ask the client to describe history of problems in bone, muscle, or joint function, including history of recent falls, trauma, lifting heavy objects, and bone or joint disease with sudden or gradual onset. In addition, have clients point out the locations of alterations.
- Assess the nature and extent of any stiffness or pain, including location, duration, severity, type of pain, and predisposing, aggravating, and relieving factors.
- Ask whether the client has noticed a change in ability to perform self-care tasks, such as bathing, feeding, dressing, voiding, and ambulating, or social functions, such as household chores, work, recreation, and sexual activities.

General Inspection

Assessment	Normal Findings
Observe the client's gait, stance, and posture from the time the assessment begins, when the client is more likely to be natural in posture and movements.	Client should normally walk with arms swinging freely at sides and head leading the body. Toes should point straight ahead.
Ask the client to walk in a straight line away from you and return; observe movement of extremities.	

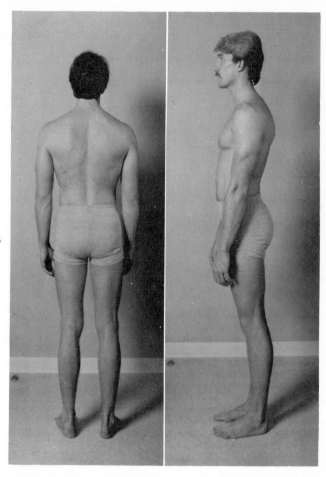

Fig. 48

A, Normal standing position. Client's hips and shoulders are aligned and parallel. **B,** Viewing the client sideways allows the examiner to observe cervical, thoracic, and lumbar curves.

(From Potter PA and Perry AG: Fundamentals of nursing: concepts, process, and practice, ed 2, St Louis, 1989, The CV Mosby Co.)

Assessment	Normal Findings
Note any foot dragging, limping, shuffling, and note the position of the trunk in relation to the legs.	
Observe client from side in a standing position and assess cervical, thoracic, and lumbar spinal curves (Fig. 48).	Normal standing posture is upright with hips and shoulders in parallel alignment. The head is normally held erect.
Also note base of support and weight-bearing stability.	Some shoulder rounding when sitting is normal. Weight is evenly distributed; the client stands on right and left heels and toes.

Range of Joint Motion and Muscle Tone and Strength
Assessment techniques

Assessment	Normal Findings
Table 14 defines terminology for normal range of joint motion positions.	
Put each joint through its full range of motion, following these general principles:	Table 15 lists the normal range of motion for all joints.
If the client is weakened by illness, assess range of joint motion with passive movement.	Joints should be free of stiffness, instability, swelling, or inflammation.
Compare the same joints on both sides for equality.	
Do not force any joint into a painful position.	*Text continued on p. 222.*

Table 14   Terminology for normal range of joint motion positions

Term	Range of Motion	Example of Joints
Flexion	Movement decreases the angle between two adjoining bones; bending of a limb	Elbow, finger, and knee
Extension	Movement increases the angle between two adjoining bones	Elbow, finger, and knee
Hyperextension	Moving a body part beyond its normal resting extended position	Head
Pronation	Front or ventral surface of a body part faces downward	Hand and forearm
Supination	Front or ventral surface of a body part faces upward	Hand and forearm
Abduction	Movement of an extremity away from the midline of the body	Leg, arm, and finger
Adduction	Movement of an extremity toward the midline of the body	Leg, arm, and finger
Internal rotation	Rotation of a joint inward	Knee and hip
External rotation	Rotation of a joint outward	Knee and hip
Eversion	Turning of the body part away from the midline	Foot
Inversion	Turning of the body part toward the midline	Foot
Dorsiflexion	Flexion of the toes and foot upward	Foot
Plantar flexion	Bending of the toes and foot downward	Foot

Table 15   Normal range of joint motion

Body Part	Motion	Measurement
Jaw	Open and close jaw	Able to insert three fingers
	Move jaw from side to side	Bottom side teeth overlap top side teeth
	Move jaw forward	Top teeth fall behind lower teeth
Neck	Touch chin to sternum	Flexion 70°–90°
	Extend neck with chin pointing toward ceiling	Hyperextension 55°
	Bend neck laterally, ear toward shoulder	Lateral bending 35°
	Rotation of neck with ear toward chest	Rotate 70° to the left and right
Spine	Bend forward at the waist	Flexion 75°
	Bend backward	Extension 30°
	Bend to each side	Lateral bending 35°
Shoulder	Abduct arm straight up	Abduction 180°
	Adduct arm toward midline of trunk	Adduction 45°
	Abduct arm straight horizontally to floor; bring arm backward toward spine and forward across chest	Horizontal extension 45° / Horizontal flexion 130°
	Forward flexion or elevation with arm straight	Flexion 180°
	Backward extension with arm straight	Extension 60°
Elbow	Extend lower arm to normal extreme	Extension 150°
	Flex lower arm toward biceps	Flexion 150°
	Hyperextend arm beyond normal resting point	Hyperextension 0°–10°

Continued.

Table 15   Normal range of joint motion—cont'd

Body Part	Motion	Measurement
Elbow	Supinate lower arm	Supination 90°
	Pronate lower arm	Pronation 90°
Wrist	Flex wrist toward lower arm	Flexion 80°-90°
	Extend wrist backward	Extension 70°
	Deviate wrist laterally toward radius	Radial deviation 20°
	Deviate wrist laterally toward ulna	Ulnar deviation 30°-50°
Fingers	Flex fingers into a fist and then extend them flat	Flexion 80°-100° (varies with joint)
		Extension 0°-45°
	Spread fingers apart	Abduction 20° between fingers
	Cross fingers together	Adduction (fingers touch)
	Opposition—able to touch each fingertip with thumb	Includes abduction, rotation, and flexion
Hip	Raise leg with knee straight	Flexion 90°
	Raise leg with knee flexed	Flexion 110°120°
	Lying prone, extend leg straight back	Extension 30°
	Abduct partially flexed leg outward	Abduction 45°-50°
	Adduct partially flexed leg inward	Adduction 20°-30°
	Flex knee and swing foot away from midline	Internal rotation 35°-40°
	Flex knee and swing foot toward midline	External rotation 45°

Knee	Flex knee with calf touching thigh	Flexion 130°
	Extend knee beyond normal point of extension	Hyperextension 15°
	Rotate knee and lower leg toward midline	Internal rotation 10°
Ankle	Dorsiflex foot with toes pointing toward head	Dorsiflexion 20°
	Plantar flex foot with toes pointing down	Plantar flexion 45°
	Turn foot away from midline	Eversion 20°
	Turn foot toward midline	Inversion 30°
Toes	Curl toes under foot	Flexion 35°-60° (varies with joints)
	Raise toes to point upward	Extension 0°-90° (varies with joints)
	Toes spread apart	Varies

Assessment	Normal Findings
Throughout the range of motion and muscle tone and strength assessments, inspect for swelling, deformity, and condition of surrounding tissues; palpate or observe for stiffness, instability, unusual joint movement, tenderness, pain, and nodules.	Normal joints move freely without tenderness or crepitation.
If a joint appears swollen and inflamed, palpate for warmth.	
If joint motion reduction is suspected, use a goniometer for precise measurement of the degree of joint movement:	
Measure the joint angle before range of motion and again after moving the joint (Fig. 49).	
Compare findings with normal degree of joint movement.	
Muscle tone and strength can be assessed during measurement of range of motion.	Normal muscle tone causes a mild, even resistance to passive movement throughout the range of motion.
Tone is detected as a slight muscular resistance as relaxed extremity is passively moved through range of motion.	
Examine each muscle group in the following manner to assess muscle strength and compare both sides:	The dominant-side arm is normally stronger than the nondominant-side arm.
Have client assume a stable position. Ask the client to perform maneuvers that demonstrate the strength of major muscle groups (Table 16).	

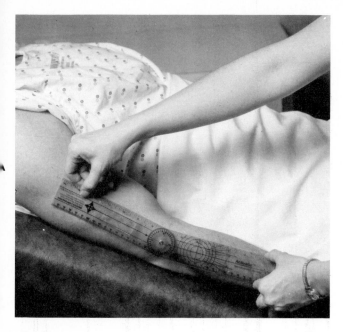

Fig. 49
A, Position goniometer at center of elbow with arms extending along client's upper and lower arms.   *Continued.*

Assessment	Normal Findings
With each maneuver: Have the client assume a position of strength. Apply a gradual increase in pressure to muscle group. Client resists pressure by attempting to move the joint against the pressure. Client maintains resistance until asked to stop. Joint should move as examiner varies the amount of pressure applied against the muscle group.	

B

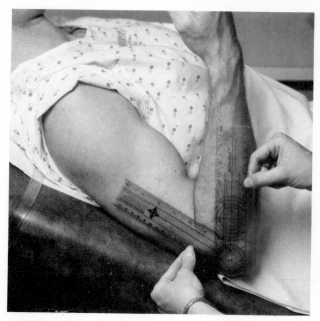

Fig. 49, cont'd.
B, After client flexes arm, goniometer measures degree of joint flexion.
(From Potter PA and Perry AG: Fundamentals of nursing: concepts, process, and practice, ed 2, St Louis, 1989, The CV Mosby Co.)

Assessment	Normal Findings
If muscle weakness is noted, measure muscle size by placing a tape measure around muscle body's circumference and compare with opposite side.	

Deviations from Normal

Gait abnormalities include foot dragging, limping, shuffling, and abnormal position of trunk in relation to legs.

Table 16   Maneuvers to assess muscle strength

Muscle Group	Maneuver
Neck (sternocleidomastoid)	Place hand firmly against the client's upper jaw. Ask the client to turn head laterally against resistance.
Shoulder (trapezius)	Place hand over midline of the client's shoulder, exerting firm pressure. Have the client raise shoulders against resistance.
Elbow	
Biceps	Pull down on the forearm as the client attempts to flex arm.
Triceps	As the client's arm is flexed, apply pressure against the forearm. Ask the client to straighten the arm.
Hip	
Quadriceps	With the client sitting, apply downward pressure to the thigh. Ask the client to raise leg up from table.
Gastrocnemius	Client sits. Hold the shin of a flexed leg and ask the client to straighten leg against resistance.

Deviations from Normal

Postural abnormalities include kyphosis (hunched back, exaggerated posterior curve of thoracic spine), lordosis (swayback or increased lumbar curvature), and scoliosis (lateral spinal curvature).

Range of motion abnormalities:

Instability or stiffness in a joint.

Unusual movement felt in a joint.

Swollen or inflamed joints or warmth in a joint on palpation.

Muscle atrophy and skin changes surrounding the joint.

Nurse Alert

Abnormalities may require special positioning techniques for clients for whom bedrest is prescribed.

Active or passive range of motion exercises are necessary for clients with partial or full immobilization.

Deviations from Normal	Nurse Alert
Range of motion significantly less than normal (Table 15).	
With increased muscle tone or hypertonicity, any sudden passive joint movement meets significant resistance.	
Hypotonic tone causes the muscle to feel flabby, and the extremity hangs loosely.	
A muscle that is atrophied or reduced in size may feel soft and boggy on palpation.	

Nursing Diagnosis

Assessment data may reveal the following nursing diagnoses:
- Pain related to joint inflammation.
- Impaired physical mobility related to pain and muscular weakness.
- Self-care deficit related to impaired upper extremity mobility.
- Potential for injury related to unsteady gait.

Pediatric Considerations

- In the neonate the spine is gently rounded rather than the characteristic S shape. Hyperflexibility of the joints is characteristic of Down syndrome.
- An infant has a bowlegged pattern until 18 to 24 months of age.
- Toddlers usually have a wide-based gait until 2 years of age.

Gerontologic Considerations

- The older adult fatigues easily, has a slower reaction time as a result of a decrease in nerve conduction and muscle tone, and may not display smooth, coordinated movement. Allow clients in this age-group adequate time for rest during the physical examination.
- Elderly clients walk with smaller steps and a wider base of support.

- Clients lose height because intervertebral space narrows.
- Range of motion is limited.
- Kyphosis is common in elderly clients.

Client Teaching

- Instruct the client about correct posture. Consult with a physical therapist about exercises to improve the client's posture.
- To reduce bone demineralization, instruct the client on a proper exercise program, for example, walking, to be followed three or more times a week. Also encourage intake of calcium to meet the recommended daily allowance.
- Instruct the client on the use of assistive devices such as zippers on clothing instead of buttons, elevated chairs to minimize bending of hips and knees, and use of crutches and walkers.
- Instruct the elderly to pace activities to compensate for loss in muscle strength.
- Discuss pain relief measures such as relaxation, massage, distraction, and heat applications.
- For clients with an unstable gait discuss safety precautions in the home such as removal of throw rugs and installation of grab bars alongside stairs.

Neurologic System

24

Assessment of the neurologic system includes assessing the following areas, described separately in the following sections: mental and emotional status, cranial nerve function, sensory function, motor function, and reflexes. Full assessment of neurologic functions can be time consuming, but neurologic measurements can be integrated with other parts of the physical examination; for example, mental and emotional status can be observed while taking the nursing history, and reflexes can be measured while the musculoskeletal system is assessed.

The examiner first decides how complete the neurologic assessment should be, based on the purpose of the assessment and the client's complaint. If the client complains of recurrent headaches or loss of function in an extremity, for example, complete neurologic assessment is required. For a complaint of abdominal pain or difficulty in breathing, on the other hand, only brief neurologic screening is necessary.

The extent of the neurologic assessment may also be limited by client factors. For example, the client's level of consciousness may limit the ability to follow directions, or physical weakness or immobility may limit the testing of coordination or reflexes.

Anatomy and Physiology

The neurologic system is responsible for many functions, including initiation and coordination of movement, reception and perception of sensory stimuli, organization of thought processes, control of speech, and storage of memory. The neurologic system is closely integrated with all other body systems.

Rationale

The integrity of the nervous system is necessary for the function of almost all bodily functions. The nurse's assessment primarily focuses on a client's sensory, motor, affective, and intellectual capacities. Disturbances in any of these functions may make clients incapable of caring for themselves and often place them at significant risk for further injury. Neurologic deficits can have an impact on a client's self-concept and create a significant threat to the life-style of clients and their family members.

Neurologic Assessment
Special Equipment

The following equipment is used to assess the neurologic system:
Reading material
Vials containing aromatic substances (for example, vanilla and coffee)
Safety pins (sterile)
Snellen chart
Penlight
Vials containing sugar or salt
Tongue blade
Two test tubes—one filled with hot water, and one filled with cold water
Cotton balls or cotton-tipped applicators
Tuning fork
Reflex hammer

Client Preparation

- During the mental and emotional assessment, a client may assume a comfortable sitting or lying position.
- A client sits during cranial nerve assessment.
- Assessment of sensory, motor, and reflex function can require the client to assume various positions.

History

- Determine whether the client is taking analgesics, sedatives, hypnotics, antipsychotics, antidepressants, or nervous system stimulants.
- Screen the client for headaches, seizures, tremors, dizziness, vertigo, numbness or tingling of a body part, visual changes, weakness, pain, or changes in speech.
- Discuss with the client's spouse, family members, or friends any recent changes in the client's behavior, for example, increased irritability, mood swings, or memory loss.

- The examiner should ask about the client's history of changes in vision, hearing, smell, taste, or touch.

Mental and Emotional Status

Assessment of emotional and mental status includes the client's level of consciousness, behavior and appearance, language, and intellectual function, including memory, knowledge, abstract thinking capabilities, association, and judgment.

Much of this assessment can be accomplished through general interaction with the client throughout other parts of the assessment by posing questions and remaining observant of the client at all times to determine appropriateness of emotions and thoughts expressed.

To ensure an objective assessment the nurse must consider the client's cultural and educational background, values, beliefs, previous experiences, and current level of coping.

Assessment	Normal Findings
Level of consciousness:	
Converse with a client, asking questions about events or activities occurring around the client or concerns about any health problems.	Fully conscious clients respond to questions quickly and are perceptive of events around them.
As consciousness lowers, use the Glasgow Coma Scale (Table 17) to measure consciousness objectively. Be sure client is fully alert before beginning.	The client normally responds cooperatively to the examiner's instructions throughout the assessment.

Nurse Alert

Be cautious in using scale if client has a sensory loss such as hearing, vision, or both. The higher the score on the coma scale, the more normal is the level of functioning.

Table 17   Glasgow coma scale

Action	Response	Score*
Eyes open	Spontaneously	4
	To speech	3
	To pain	2
	None	1
Best verbal response	Oriented	5
	Confused	4
	Inappropriate words	3
	Incomprehensible sounds	2
	None	1
Best motor response	Obeys command	6
	Localized pain	5
	Flexion withdrawal	4
	Abnormal flexion	3
	Abnormal extension	2
	Flaccid	1

*Total score of best possible responses is 15.

Assessment	Normal Findings
Ask short simple questions such as "What is your name?" or "Where are you?" Ask the client to follow simple commands such as "Squeeze my fingers."	
If the client's consciousness is lowered to the point of no apparent responsiveness, attempt to elicit a response by applying firm pressure with thumb to fingernail or area over the sternum.	Normal response to painful stimulus is withdrawal of body part from stimulus.

Assessment	Normal Findings

Behavior and appearance:

During initial general survey note the client's hygiene, grooming, and clothing.

Observe the client's mannerisms and actions throughout the assessment, noting nonverbal, as well as verbal, behaviors.

Consider these questions:

Does the client respond appropriately to directions?

Does the client's mood vary with no apparent cause?

Normally the client shows some degree of personal hygiene.

Choice and fit of clothing may reflect socioeconomic background or personal taste rather than indicate deficient self-concept or poor judgment.

Clothing should be appropriate for type of weather.

Client follows directions, maintains good eye contact, and expresses self clearly.

Language:

When it is clear that communication with a client is ineffective, assess for evidence of aphasia:

Ask the client to name familiar objects when the nurse points at them.

Client names objects correctly.

Ask the client to respond to simple verbal and written commands such as "stand up" or "sit down."

Client can follow commands.

Ask the client to read simple sentences out loud.

Client reads sentences correctly.

Assessment	Normal Findings

Intellectual function:

Avoid threatening the client or making the client feel uncomfortable. Using a casual manner ask questions about concepts or ideas with which the client is familiar.

Assess recall and recent and remote memory.

Test immediate recall by asking client to repeat a series of numbers in the order they are presented or in reverse order.

People normally can recall five to eight digits in the presented order or four to six digits in reverse order.

Gradually increase the number of digits until the client fails to repeat the digits correctly.

Test recent memory by asking client to recall events occurring during the same day, for example, what was eaten for breakfast and what kind of transportation the client used to come to the hospital. Confirm the client's answers with family or friends.

Client recalls events readily.

Ask the client to recall information shared earlier such as the name of a nurse.

Assessment	Normal Findings
Test remote memory by asking client to recall things such as medical history, family history, anniversaries, or birthdays. Ask open-ended questions rather than simple yes/no questions.	Client should have immediate recall of such information.
Assess a client's knowledge and ability to learn and understand by asking about such things as the client's illness or state of health and reason for hospitalization.	
Assess the client's capacity for abstract thinking by asking for an interpretation of a saying, such as "An ounce of prevention is worth a pound of cure."	The client's explanations of common sayings show abstract thought processes by their relevancy and perceptiveness. The client normally can make judgments and associations consistent with experience and level of intelligence.
Assess the client's associational thinking with concept association questions such as: "A collie is to a dog as a Siamese is to a what?" Questions should be appropriate to the client's level of intelligence.	
Assess the client's ability to make judgments and to organize thoughts with questions such as "Why did you decide to seek health care?" or "What would you do if you suddenly became ill while home alone?"	Client can make logical decisions.

Deviations from Normal	Nurse Alert

Alterations in mental or emotional status may be caused by disturbances in cerebral functioning related to pathologic conditions of the brain, drug effects, or metabolic changes.

Alterations in level of consciousness may be manifested as the following (in order of increasing alteration):
Irritability, short attention span, or dulled perception or environment.
Disorientation.
Inability to recall name or time of day.
Inability to follow even simple commands such as "Move your toes."

Responsive only to painful stimuli.
Completely unresponsive to verbal and painful stimuli (comatose).

Severe emotional stress may cause confusion and disorientation.
Inappropriate clothing for the weather may indicate reduced mental status.
Deterioration in appearance may be caused by a poor self-image or inability to consciously attend to grooming.

The client's ability to understand and answer questions has implications for the remainder of the neurologic examination and other parts of the physical assessment: the examiner may have to skip or delay parts of the examination that require feedback if the client is confused or irritable.

Disorientation or confusion may result from any of the following physiologic causes: pain, fever, substance abuse, electrolyte imbalance, side or toxic effects of medications, circulatory shock, severe anemia, hypoxia, diabetic coma, or liver failure. Any sudden change in responsiveness or orientation requires immediate notification of the physician.

Deviations from Normal	Nurse Alert
A client with reduced mentation may be unable to interpret or understand questions requiring abstract thinking or may react by merely paraphrasing the words or interpreting the words too literally.	

Nursing Diagnosis

Assessment data may reveal the following nursing diagnoses:
- Impaired verbal communication related to expressive aphasia.
- Altered thought processes related to physiologic changes.

Pediatric Considerations

- Parents should act as resources for information regarding any recent change in child's behavior, attention span, or school performance.

Gerontologic Considerations

- The older adult may need additional time to respond to questions requiring the use of memory, judgment, or other cognitive functions.
- Commonly elderly clients show symptoms of confusion and forgetfulness resulting from normal neurologic changes. Sudden confusion, however, is usually unrelated to age. The elderly client is at greater risk of confusion from acute conditions such as dehydration, infection, drug toxicity, or hypoglycemia.

Client Teaching

- Explain to the client's family and friends the implications of any mental impairment shown by the client.

Cranial Nerve Assessment

The function of each of the 12 cranial nerves should be assessed. Table 18 describes the function and assessment method for each nerve. An inability to perform any of these activities may indicate a cranial nerve alteration.

Table 18   Cranial nerve function and assessment

Nerve	Function	Action	Method of Assessment
I Olfactory	Sensory	Smell	Ask client to identify different nonirritating aromas such as coffee or vanilla
II Optic	Sensory	Vision	Snellen chart; ask client to read printed material
III Oculomotor	Motor	Extraocular eye movement; pupil constriction and dilation	Assess directions of gaze; measure pupil reaction to light reflex
IV Trochlear	Motor	Upward and downward movement of eyeball	Assess directions of gaze
V Trigeminal	Sensory and motor	Sensory nerve to skin of face; motor nerve to muscles of jaw	Assess corneal reflex; measure sensation of light, touch, and pain across skin of face; assess client's ability to clench teeth by palpating masseter and temporal muscles
VI Abducens	Motor	Lateral movement of eyeballs	Assess directions of gaze
VII Facial	Sensory and motor	Facial expression	Ask client to smile, frown, puff out cheeks, and raise and lower eyebrows

Continued.

Table 18 Cranial nerve function and assessment—cont'd

Nerve	Function	Action	Method of Assessment
VII Facial		Taste	Have client identify salty or sweet tastes on front of tongue
VIII Auditory	Sensory	Hearing	Assess client's ability to hear spoken word
IX Glossopharyngeal	Sensory and motor	Taste; ability to swallow; movement of tongue	Ask client to identify sour, salty, or sweet taste on back of tongue; use tongue blade to elicit gag reflex; ask client to move tongue
X Vagus	Sensory and motor	Sensation of pharynx; ability to swallow; movement of vocal cords	Ask client to say "ah"; observe palatal and pharyngeal movement; use tongue blade to elicit gag reflex; assess client's speech for hoarseness
XI Spinal accessory	Motor	Movement of head and shoulders	Ask client to shrug shoulders and turn head against examiner's passive resistance
XII Hypoglossal	Motor	Position of tongue	Ask client to stick out tongue to the midline

Deviations From Normal

Inability to identify aroma.

Abnormalities related to optic, oculomotor, trochlear, and abducens
nerve dysfunction are summarized in Chapter 12.

Inability to identify or feel sensation in face.

Inability to smile symmetrically.

Absent or one-sided blinking of eyelids and raising of eyebrows.

Irregular and unequal facial movements.

Inability to taste or identify taste.

Inability to hear spoken word.

Unequal or absent rise of uvula and soft palate as the client says
"ah".

Absent gag reflex.

Tongue deviation to side.

Weak or absent shoulder and neck movement.

Nursing Diagnosis

Assessment data may reveal the following nursing diagnosis:
- Sensory/perceptual alterations (auditory, gustatory, tactile, olfactory) related to neurologic injury.

Gerontologic Considerations

- See Chapters 12 and 13 regarding the elderly client's limitations resulting from visual and hearing impairment.
- Atrophy of the taste buds is normal in elderly clients.

Client Teaching

See Chapters 12 and 13 regarding instructions for clients with
hearing and vision loss.

Sensory Nerve Function Assessment

A quick screening of sensory function is sufficient for most clients unless there are symptoms of altered or decreased sensation,
motor impairment, or paralysis.

The sensory pathways of the central nervous system conduct
sensations of pain, temperature, position, vibration, and crude
and finely localized touch.

Assessment	Normal Findings
Perform all sensory testing with the client's eyes closed.	Clients normally have sensory response to all the stimuli tested.
Apply stimuli in random unpredictable order to maintain the client's attention.	Sensations are felt equally on both sides of the body in all areas.
Ask the client to tell you when and where each stimulus is perceived.	
Compare symmetric areas of body for response to stimuli.	
Table 19 lists the specific tests of sensory function.	
If a deficit is found, map it out carefully to measure the extent of impairment.	

Deviations from Normal

Any deviation from normal sensory response may result from peripheral nerve alterations, such as from localized edema, reduced blood flow, trauma, and pressure from tumor, or from altered spinal cord function. Peripheral nerve alterations produce local alterations; spinal cord alterations produce more regional or widespread alterations.

Nursing Diagnosis

Assessment data may reveal the following nursing diagnoses:
- Sensory/perceptual alteration (tactile) related to neurologic trauma.
- Potential for injury related to paresthesia.

Gerontologic Considerations

- Conduction velocity in peripheral nerves declines with age.
- The tactile sense is blunted, and therefore more intense stimuli are required to test this sense.
- Proprioception in the older adult becomes increasingly less functional with age.
- Elderly clients have reduced pain sensation bilaterally.

Table 19 Assessment of sensory nerve function

Sensory Function	Equipment	Method	Precautions
Pain	Safety pin	Ask client to tell you when a dull or sharp sensation is felt. Alternately apply the pointed and blunt ends of the pin to the skin's surface. Note areas of numbness or increased sensitivity.	Areas where skin is thickened, such as heel or sole of foot, may be less sensitive to pain.
Temperature	Two test tubes; one filled with hot water, the other with cold water	Touch the client's skin with the tube. Ask the client to identify hot versus cold sensation.	May omit test if pain sensation is normal.
Light touch	Cotton ball or cotton-tipped applicator	Apply a light wisp of cotton to different points along the skin surface. Ask the client to tell you when a sensation is felt.	Apply cotton along areas where the client's skin is thin or more sensitive, such as the face, neck, inner aspect of arms, or top of feet and hands.
Vibration	Tuning fork	Apply vibrating fork to distal interphalangeal joint of fingers and interphalangeal joint of the great toe.	Be sure the client feels vibration and not merely pressure. Have the client tell you when the vibration stops.

Continued.

Table 19   Assessment of sensory nerve function—cont'd

Sensory Function	Equipment	Method	Precautions
Position		Grasp the client's finger, holding it by its sides with your thumb and index finger. Alternate moving the finger up and down. Ask the client to tell you whether the finger is up or down. Repeat procedure with the toes.	Avoid rubbing adjacent appendages as the finger or toe is moved.
Two-point discrimination	Two safety pins	Lightly apply the points of the safety pins simultaneously to the skin's surface. Ask the client if one or two pinpricks are felt.	Apply pins to same anatomic site, for example, the fingertips, palm of hand, upper arms, or back. Minimum distance at which a client can discriminate two points varies (normally 2 or 3 mm apart on fingertips, 40 to 70 mm apart on back).

Client Teaching

- Explain measures to ensure the client's safety, for example, using caution when applying ice packs or heating pads.
- Teach elderly clients to observe skin surfaces for areas of trauma, since pain perception is reduced.

Motor Function

Motor function assessment includes measurements performed in the musculoskeletal assessment and a review of cerebellar function.

Assessment	Normal Findings
To assess musculoskeletal function see Chapter 23.	
To test coordination, demonstrate each of the following maneuvers to the client and ask the client to repeat them, observing for smoothness and balance in the client's movements.	
Close eyes and hold both arms straight and over the head for 20 seconds.	Arms remain in steady position.
With arms extended out to sides, touch each forefinger alternately to the nose (first with eyes open, then with eyes closed).	Client can alternately touch nose smoothly.
In sitting position, pat hand against thigh as fast as possible.	Client should be able to strike thigh rapidly and without hesitation.
Pat thigh as fast as possible with hand alternately supinated and pronated.	The client's dominant hand is normally less awkward in coordinated movements.
Touch each finger with the thumb of the same hand in rapid sequence.	Client should be able to touch each finger with the thumb of the same hand smoothly in succession.

Assessment	Normal Findings
With client supine, place your hand at ball of client's foot and ask client to tap your hand with the foot as quickly as possible, observing each foot for speed and smoothness.	The feet are not as rapid or as even in coordinated movements as are the hands.
With client sitting with eyes closed, ask client to place heel of foot on opposite knee and then slide the heel down the leg to the foot.	Client normally can slide the heel from knee to foot without the heel sliding off the leg.
To assess balance, have client stand with feet together and eyes open, then ask the client to close eyes to test for Romberg sign. Note any swaying and protect the client from falling.	Client does not normally have to break stance to maintain balance.
A further test of balance involves having the client close the eyes and stand on one foot and then the other.	

Deviations From Normal

Arms drift downward while client attempts to hold them straight out.

Inability to touch nose, uncoordinated movement.

Client hesitates striking thigh or touching fingers; movements are awkward.

Unable to place heel on knee or move it down leg.

Client sways and moves feet to stop a fall.

Nursing Diagnosis

Assessment data may reveal the following nursing diagnoses:

- Altered physical mobility related to incoordination.
- Potential for injury related to incoordination.

Gerontologic Considerations

- A normally slow reaction time may cause movements to be less rhythmic in elderly clients.

- Slight swaying when the client stands with feet together and eyes closed is normal for an elderly client.

Client Teaching

- Explain safety measures such as the use of ambulation aids or the use of safety bars in bathrooms or stairways.

Reflexes

Eliciting reflex reactions allows the nurse to assess the integrity of sensory and motor pathways of the reflex arc and specific spinal cord segments. Testing does not determine higher neural center functioning.

When the muscle and tendon are stretched during a reflex test, nerve impulses travel along afferent nerve pathways to the dorsal horn of the spinal cord segment. Impulses synapse and travel to the efferent motor neuron in the spinal cord. A motor nerve then sends the impulses back to the muscle, causing the reflex response.

Client Preparation

Help the client relax and avoid voluntary movement or tensing of muscles. Position extremities to slightly stretch the muscle being tested.

Assessment Techniques

Assessment	Normal Findings
Table 20 lists common deep tendon and cutaneous reflexes.	
Hold reflex hammer loosely to allow it to swing freely to tap the tendon briskly (Figure 50). Compare symmetry of reflexes on both sides of body	Reflex response is brisk. Record reflex findings on a scale of 0 to 4: 0—no response 1—low normal or diminished response 2—normal 3—brisker than normal 4—hyperactive and very brisk (may be associated with spinal cord disorder)

Table 20 Common reflexes

Type	Procedure	Normal Reflex
Deep Tendon Reflexes		
Biceps	Flex the client's arm at the elbow with palms down. Place your thumb in the antecubital fossa at the base of the biceps tendon. Strike the thumb with the reflex hammer.	Flexion of arm at elbow
Triceps	Flex the client's elbow, holding the arm across the chest, or hold the upper arm horizontally and allow the lower arm to go limp. Strike the triceps tendon, just above the elbow.	Extension at elbow
Patellar	Have the client sit with legs hanging freely over the side of the bed or chair or have the client lie supine and support knee in a flexed position. Briskly tap the patellar tendon just below the patella.	Extension of lower leg at knee

Achilles	Have the client assume the same position as for patellar reflex. Slightly dorsiflex the client's ankle by grasping the toes in the palm of your hand and turning them upward. Strike Achilles tendon just above the heel.	Bending of toes downward
Plantar (Babinski)	Have the client lie supine with legs straight and feet relaxed. Take the handle end of the reflex hammer and stroke the lateral aspect of the sole from the heel to the ball of the foot, curving across the ball.	Flexion of the toes
Cutaneous Reflexes Gluteal	Have the client assume a side lying position. Spread apart the client's buttocks and lightly stimulate the perineal area with a cotton-tipped applicator.	Contraction of anal sphincter

Continued.

Table 20 Common reflexes-cont'd

Type	Procedure	Normal Reflex
Abdominal	Have the client stand or lie supine. Stroke the abdominal skin with the base of a cotton-tipped applicator over the lateral borders of the rectus abdominal muscles toward the midline. Repeat the test in each abdominal quadrant.	Rectus abdominal muscles contract with pulling of umbilicus toward the stimulated side
Cremasteric	Stroke the inner upper thigh of the male client, using a cotton-tipped applicator.	Scrotum elevates on stimulated side.

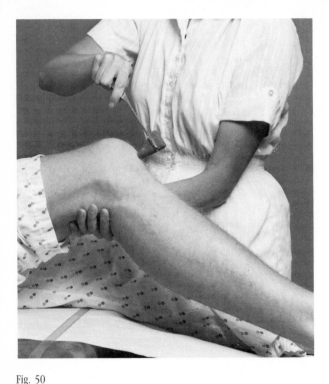

Fig. 50
Position for eliciting patellar tendon reflex.
(From Potter PA and Perry AG: Fundamentals of nursing: concepts, process, and practice, ed 2, St Louis, 1989, The CV Mosby Co.)

Assessment	Normal Findings
If necessary, distract the client during testing to increase reflex response by asking the client to clench teeth while testing upper extremities or asking the client to interlock hands and pull outward while testing upper extremities.	

Deviations From Normal

Absent or hyperactive reflex response of deep tendons.

Abnormal Babinski sign, that is, extension of great toe with all other toes fanning out.

No abdominal contraction during cutaneous reflex test.

No elevation of scrotum during a cremasteric test.

Pediatric Considerations

There are a number of reflexes to assess an infant's developmental status including the following:

Rooting reflex — infant turns head toward side of face stroked (disappears at 3 to 12 months of age)

Grasp reflex — infant flexes the hand or toes when light touch is applied to the palm of the hand or the sole of the foot (disappears at 3 months of age)

Moro reflex — sudden jarring of infant while lying down causes infant to suddenly extend and abduct extremities. Crying also is elicited (disappears at 3 to 4 months of age)

Dance reflex — infant is held upright so that the feet touch a flat surface to stimulate walking movement (disappears at 3 to 4 weeks of age)

Gerontologic Considerations

■ Reflexes are normally slowed in elderly clients.

Completing the Examination

25

The following is a list of those things to be done at the completion of the examination:

Help the client dress if necessary.

If desired, provide client with a clean gown and the opportunity for personal hygiene.

Help the hospital client return to bed and assume a comfortable position.

Share a summary of the assessment findings with the client along with any final teaching activities.

If the findings suggest a serious abnormality such as a tumor or seriously irregular heartbeat, consult with the physician before revealing findings to the client.

Clean the examination area: store reusable equipment, dispose of used nonreusable supplies, clean the bedside table, and make sure bed linen is clean and dry.

Make sure assessment recording is complete.

Review entries made during the examination for accuracy and thoroughness.

Communicate significant findings to appropriate medical and nursing personnel.

Recording and Reporting the Physical Assessment Findings

- The general characteristics of quality reporting and recording are:

    Accuracy
    Conciseness
    Thoroughness
    Currentness
    Organization
    Confidentiality

- Immediately following the physical assessment, while your memory is still current, review all data recorded on the assessment form to ensure that all notes are legible, to complete any sections not yet filled in, and to clarify any potentially unclear findings or observations.
- Any abnormal assessment findings should be directly reported to other appropriate health care professionals, depending on the seriousness and urgency of need for intervention, in addition to recording the findings on the assessment form.
- Review all available assessment data and select appropriate care plans based on the nursing diagnoses identified for the client.

Bibliography

American Nurses Association: Social policy statement 1980, Kansas City, Mo, 1980, The Association.

American Cancer Society: 1989 cancer facts and figures, New York, 1989, The Society.

American Cancer Society: Guidelines for the cancer-related checkup: recommendations and rationale, New York, 1980, The Society.

Assessing your patients: 1982 nursing photobook, Springhouse, Pa, 1982, Intermed Communications, Inc.

Bates B: A guide to physical examination, ed 4, Philadelphia, 1987, JB Lippincott Co.

Becker KL and Stevens SA: Performing in-depth abdominal assessment, Nursing 18(6):59, 1988.

Berliner H: Aging skin, I, Am J Nurs 86:1138, 1986.

Berliner H: Aging skin, II, Am J Nurs 86:1259, 1986.

Blair JD: A quick, high-yield mouth exam, Patient Care 19:33, 1985.

Block G et al: Health assessment for professional nursing, New York, 1981, Appleton-Century-Crofts.

Bowers A and Thompson J: Clinical manual of health assessment, St Louis, 1984, The CV Mosby Co.

Brown MC, Brown JD, and Boyer MM: Changing nursing practice through continuing education in physical assessment: perceived barriers to implementation, J Contin Educ Nurs 18(4):111, 1987.

Bulau J: Clinical policies and procedures for home health care, Rockville, Md, 1986, Aspen Publishers Inc.

Burger D: Breast self-examination, Am J Nurs 79:1088, 1979.

Burggraf V and Donlon B: Assessing the elderly, system by system, Am J Nurs 85:974, 1985.

Calvani D: Assessing the elderly, II, Am J Nurs 85:1103, 1985.

Casey MP: Testicular cancer: the worst disease at the worst time, RN 50:36, 1987.

Church JC and Baer KJ: Examination of the adolescent: a practical guide, J Pediatr Health Care 1(2):163, 1986.

Corrigan JD: Functional health pattern assessment in the emergency department, J Emerg Nurs 12(3):163, 1986.

Dennison R: Cardiopulmonary assessment, Nurs 86 16:34, 1986.

Ebersole P and Hess P: Toward healthy aging, ed 2, St Louis, 1985, The CV Mosby Co.

Erickson BA: Detecting abnormal heart sounds, Nurs 86 16:58, 1986.

Ernst ND: The national cholesterol education program's recommendations for treatment of high blood cholesterol, Fam Community Health 12:23, 1989.

Forgacs P: The functional basis of pulmonary sounds, Chest 73:399, 1978.

Fraser MC and McGuire DB: Skin cancer's early warning system, Am J Nurs 84:1232, 1984.

Gordon M: Nursing diagnosis and the diagnostic process, Am J Nurs 76:1298, 1976.

Gordon M: Nursing diagnosis, process and application, New York, 1987, McGraw-Hill Inc.

Hays AM and Borger F: Assessing the elderly: a test in-time, Am J Nurs 85:1107, 1985.

Henderson ML: Assessing the elderly: altered perception, Am J Nurs 85:1104, 1985.

Hurst JW et al: Noises in the neck, N Engl J Med 302:862, 1980.

Jacobs R: Physical changes in the aged. In Devereaux M et al, editors: Elder care: a guide to clinical geriatrics, New York, 1981, Grune & Stratton Inc.

Joint National Committee on Detection, Evaluation and Treatment of High Blood Pressure: The 1984 report of the Joint National Committee on Detection, Evaluation and Treatment of High Blood Pressure, Arch Intern Med 144:1045, 1984.

Jones D: Health assessment manual, New York, 1986, McGraw-Hill Inc.

Larson E: Evaluating validity of screening tests, Nurs Res 35:186, 1986.

Mahboub E and Sayed GM: Oral cavity and pharynx. In Schottenfeld D and Fraumeni JF Jr, editors: Cancer epidemiology and prevention, Philadelphia, 1982, WB Saunders Co.

Malkiewicz J: A pragmatic approach to musculoskeletal assessment, RN 45:56, 1982.

McFarland GK: Nursing diagnosis: the critical link in the nursing process. In McFarland GK and McFarland EA, editors: Nursing diagnosis and intervention, St Louis, 1989, The CV Mosby Co.

Merry JA: Take your assessment all the way down to the toes, RN 51(11):60, 1988.

Miracle VA: Anatomy of a murmur, Nurs 86 16:26, 1986.

Miracle VA: Get in touch and in tune with cardiac assessment, Nurs 1988 18(4):41, 1988.

Norman S: The pupil check, Am J Nurs 82:588, 1982.

Phipps W et al: Medical-surgical nursing: concepts and clinical practice, ed 3, St Louis, 1987, The CV Mosby Co.

Potter PA and Perry AG: Fundamentals of nursing: concepts, process, and practice, ed 2, St Louis, 1989, The CV Mosby Co.

Reynolds JI and Logsdon JB: Assessing your patients' mental status, Nurs 79 9:26, 1979.

Rutledge DN: Factors related to women's practice of breast self-examination, Nurs Res 36:117, 1987.

Sana JM and Judge RD: Physical assessment skills for nursing practice, ed 2, Boston, 1982, Little, Brown & Co Inc.

Schweiger JL et al: Oral assessment: how to do it, Am J Nurs 80:654, 1980.

Seidel HM et al: Mosby's guide to physical examination, St Louis, 1987, The CV Mosby Co.

Shoemaker J: Essential features of a nursing diagnosis. In Kim JM, McFarland G, and McLane A, editors: Classification of nursing diagnoses: proceedings of the fifth national conference, St Louis, 1984, The CV Mosby Co.

Silverberg E: Cancer statistics 1984, New York, 1984, American Cancer Society.

Smith C: Abdominal assessment: a blending of science and art, Nurs 81 11:42, 1981.

Smith CE: With good assessment skills you can construct a solid framework for patient care, Nursing 14(12):26, 1984.

Stark J: Urinary tract assessment, Nurs 88 18(7):57, 1988.

Stevens SA and Becker KL: How to perform picture-perfect respiratory assessment, Nursing 18(1):57, 1988.

Stevens S and Becker K: Neurologic assessment, I, Nurs 88 18(9):53, 1988.

Tanner JM: Growth of adolescence, ed 2, Cambridge, Mass, 1962, Blackwell Scientific Publications Inc.

Tishknobf MK: Breast cancer, the treatment evolution, Am J Nurs 84:1110, 1984.

US Department of Health and Human Services: Cancer rates and risks, ed 3, 1985, National Institute of Health.

Visich MA: Breath and heart sounds, Nurs 81 11:64, 1981.

Whaley LF and Wong DL: Nursing care of infants and children, ed 3, St Louis, 1987, The CV Mosby Co.

Wilkins RL: Lung sounds, St Louis, 1987, The CV Mosby Co.

Yacone LA: Cardiac assessment: what to do, how to do it, RN 50:42, 1987.

1983

Metropolitan
Height and
Weight Tables

1983 Metropolitan height and weight tables*

Men				
Height		Small	Medium	Large
Feet	Inches	Frame (lbs)	Frame (lbs)	Frame (lbs)
5	2	128-134	131-141	138-150
5	3	130-136	133-143	140-153
5	4	132-138	135-145	142-156
5	5	134-140	137-148	144-160
5	6	136-142	139-151	146-164
5	7	138-145	142-154	149-168
5	8	140-148	145-157	152-172
5	9	142-151	148-160	155-176
5	10	144-154	151-163	158-180
5	11	146-157	154-166	161-184
6	0	149-160	157-170	164-188
6	1	152-164	160-174	168-192
6	2	155-168	164-178	172-197
6	3	158-172	167-182	176-202
6	4	162-176	171-187	181-207

		Women		
Height		Small Frame	Medium Frame	Large Frame
Feet	Inches			
4	10	102-111	109-121	118-131
4	11	103-113	111-123	120-134
5	0	104-115	113-126	122-137
5	1	106-118	115-129	125-140
5	2	108-121	118-132	128-143
5	3	111-124	121-135	131-147
5	4	114-127	124-138	134-151
5	5	117-130	127-141	137-155
5	6	120-133	130-144	140-159
5	7	123-136	133-147	143-163
5	8	126-139	136-150	146-167
5	9	129-142	139-153	149-170
5	10	132-145	142-156	152-173
5	11	135-148	145-159	155-176
6	0	138-151	148-162	158-179

Source of basic data: 1979 Build Study, Society of Actuaries and Association of Life Insurance Medical Directors of America, 1980.

*Weights at ages 25 to 59 years based on lowest mortality. Weight in pounds according to frame (in indoor clothing weighing 5 lbs. for men and 3 lbs for women; shoes with 1″ heels).

Smooth Average Weights* for Older Men and Women

Men

Height (inches)	Weight (pounds)					
	55 to 64 Yrs	65 to 74 Yrs	75 to 79 Yrs	80 to 84 Yrs	85 to 89 Yrs	90 to 94 Yrs
62	148	144	133	135		
63	151	148	138	136	133	
64	155	151	143	138	135	
65	158	154	148	141	139	130
66	162	158	154	144	142	133
67	166	161	159	147	145	136
68	169	165	164	150	148	140
69	173	168	169	154	152	144
70	176	171	174	159	156	149
71	180	175	179	164	160	154
72	184	178	184	170	165	
73	187	182	189			
74	191	185	194			

Continued.

Height (inches)	Weight (pounds)					
	55 to 64 Yrs	65 to 74 Yrs	75 to 79 Yrs	80 to 84 Yrs	85 to 89 Yrs	90 to 94 Yrs
Women						
57	138	132	125			
58	141	135	129			
59	144	138	132			
60	149	142	136	111	110	
61	150	145	139	118	113	
62	152	149	143	121	116	
63	155	152	146	124	120	
64	158	156	150	128	124	119
65	161	159	153	132	128	119
66	164	163	157	136	133	120
67	167	166	160	140	138	124
68	170	170	164	144	142	129

Modified from Weight, height, and selected body dimensions of adults (ages 55 to 79), United States, 1960-1962. Series 11, no. 8. National Center For Health Statistics, Washington, DC; and Carnevali D and Patrick M: Nursing management for the elderly, Philadelphia, 1979, JB Lippincott Co.

*Estimated values from regression equations of weights for specific age groups.

Assessment

APPENDIX C

During

Pregnancy with

Evaluative Criteria

	First and Second Trimesters (wk 1 through 24)	Third Trimester (wk 25 through 38 to 40 [term])
Schedule of care	After initial contact and preliminary assessments, return visit scheduled for 2 wk, thereafter every 4 wk	Medical and nursing care has been increased to permit detection of any abnormal response, maternal or fetal: woman is examined every 2 wk between 32 and 36 wk and every wk between 36 and 40 wk; if indicated, plan of care is modified
Maternal Adaptations **Physical**		
Temperature	Normal range established	Normal range
Pulse	Normal range established	
Respirations	18 to 20/min	Gradual rise of +8 to +10 by 35 wk 18 to 20/min; occasional shortness of breath and sighing breaths may be troublesome at times
Blood pressure	Normal range of less than +30 systolic and +15 diastolic may decrease slightly in midpregnancy	Systolic no greater than +30 and diastolic no greater than +15 over base line, which is normally higher (+6 to +10) as term approaches
Urinalysis	Negative for protein and acetone; no greater than 1+ for glucose; negative for bacteria	Negative for protein and acetone, no greater than 1+ for glucose; lactose is present as hormone prolactin increases

Blood tests		
RBC	At sea level for wk 1 to 12: Hg, 11 g/dl; hematocrit, 37% Wk 12 to 24; Hg, 10.5 g/dl; hematocrit 35%	At sea level for wk 24 to term; Hg, 10 g/dl; hematocrit, 33% RBC repeated at 32 to 34 wk
STS (VDRL)	Negative	Negative
Weight gain	Weeks 1 to 12; about 3 to 4 lb (1.4 to 1.8 kg) Weeks 12 to 24: 12 to 14 lb (5.6 to 6.3 kg)	Wk 24 to term: no more than 1 lb (0.45 kg)/wk Approximately 24 ± 4 lb (11 kg) gain over prepregnancy weight (less than 20 lb puts fetus at risk)
	Approximately 0.5 lb (0.23 kg)/wk	
Edema	Dependent edema not yet apparent	Dependent edema of lower legs, ankles, and feet
Vagina	Bluish-red hyperemia characteristic of pregnancy, little increase in size No anomalies, including cystocele, rectocele, or relaxed perineum	Highly distensible
Cervix	Long, firm but some softening by midpregnancy	Readiness for labor Cervix becomes more softened as term approaches In parous women, external os of cervix may be about 3 cm dilated by wk 35
	Moderate white mucoid discharge	Discharge persists

Continued

From Bobak I and Jensen M: Essentials of maternity nursing, St Louis, 1983, The CV Mosby Co.

Breasts	Early weeks, breasts tender with tingling sensations	Striations may appear if increase in size of breasts extensive
	By wk 8 breasts increase in size, become nodular; veins become visible beneath skin	Areola becomes larger and more deeply pigmented and glands of Montgomery appear
	Nipples become larger, more pigmented, and more erectile	Lactogenesis begins with secretion of colostrum; may be expressed by gentle massage
	No secretions from breasts	Preparation of breasts for breastfeeding begins
Abdomen	Topic of infant feeding introduced	Enlargement continues: see height of fundus
	Gradual enlargement: see height of fundus	Toward end of pregnancy striae gravidarum may occur; in multipara glistening silvery lines of striae from earlier pregnancies may be seen
		Linea nigra at midline of abdomen
Uterus	Progressive enlargement to accommodate growing products of conception	Continued progressive enlargement of uterus

	Fundal height at 12 to 13 wk: felt just to above symphysis pubis; 16 wk: 3 to 4 cm above symphysis pubis; 20 wk: 2 to 3 cm below umbilicus; 24 wk: at umbilicus	Fundal height at 36 wk; almost to xiphoid process; 40 wk: 2 cm below because of "lightening"
		Readiness for labor: Braxton Hick's contractions may be felt by wk 34
		Pelvic measurements adequate in relation to size of fetus (examined near term)
Pelvis	Pelvis measurements within normal range (examined at second visit, not repeated) Diagonal conjugate 11.5 cm or more	
	Transverse diameter of outlet 8 cm or more	
	Ischial spines not prominent, concavity of sacrum ample, side walls of pelvis do not converge	
Skin	Changes not noticeable	May develop chloasma (mask of pregnancy), vascular spiders, palmar erythema (red palms)
		Varicose veins may appear in lower legs and vulva

Continued.

Common problems	Woman or couple verbalize understanding of physiologic basis and treatment of nausea and vomiting up to wk 12; increased skin pigmentation (for example, linea nigra); heartburn; constipation; leg cramps; pica	Woman or couple verbalize understanding of physiologic basis and treatment of hemorrhoids, varicosities, leg cramps, hypermobility of joints, backache
Abnormal symptoms	Woman or couple verbalizes understanding of physiologic basis, need for immediate treatment, and how to obtain necessary care Vaginal bleeding Burning or pain on urination Gastroenteritis Exposure to communicable disease (such as rubella) Nausea and vomiting beyond wk 12 Abdominal pain	Woman or couple verbalizes understanding of physiologic basis; need for immediate treatment and how to obtain necessary care Vaginal bleeding; at term rule ut brownish spotting occurring 8 hr after vaginal examination and/or "show" of pinkish mucus Symptoms of preeclampsia-eclampsia: weight gain over 1 lb/wk, generalized edema, persistent headache, dimness or blurring of vision Cessation, noticeable diminution, or acceleration in amount of fetal movement Rupture of membranes

Psychosocial adaptation	Reactions indicative of positive psychologic response to pregnancy, including birth process and parenthood	Burning or pain on urination
		Chills or elevated temperature
		Abdominal pain
		Persistent nausea and vomiting
	During first trimester, woman may be self-centered and concerned with her own adjustment to idea of pregnancy	Responses typical of normal findings in pregnancy
		Interest centered around preparing for parenthood
	During second trimester, woman usually is reasonably free of symptoms; she is more tranquil and at ease; reality of child is now recognized, and most women come to accept their pregnant state; however, feelings of ambivalence come and go	Anxiety may be expressed over pain of labor, behavior during labor, care of other child
	During first and second trimesters family members (spouse, others) adjust in a positive manner to the pregnancy although they may express feelings of being "left out" by mother	Ambivalent feelings persist

Continued

Psychosocial adaptation—cont'd	Verbalizes understanding of sexual responses and relates that sexual relationships are mutually accepted and serve as a means of communication	Verbalizes understanding of various modes of sexual expression (which are safe, which to avoid) and of medical acceptance of sexual intercourse with penile penetration until rupture of membranes; feelings of frustration and resentment over abstinence expressed early in third trimester and acceptance expressed in end of third trimester
	Negative feelings about self-image are recognized as temporary; expresses pride or pleasure about being pregnant	Expresses eagerness to be done with pregnancy; complaints about awkwardness, annoyance about symptoms (shortness of breath and backache) expressed; questions asked about how soon appearance will be back to "normal"
Active participation in care	Verbalizes understanding of plan of care, schedule, need for continuity of care, physical examination to be done, reporting of abnormal symptoms	Verbalizes understanding of preparation for delivery; symptoms of impending labor, including uterine contractions, rupture of membranes, and bloody "show," what to report, and where to go for delivery

Complies with care

Keeps appointments, reports abnormal symptoms promptly, follows diet plan, takes only prescribed medications, refrains from smoking and drinking alcoholic beverages, exercises

Appearance is healthy, growing adequate, energy level normal

Discusses techniques of infant feeding

Discusses prenatal education classes

Verbalizes understanding of delivery process; methods to control pain, such as analgesia, anesthesia, and breathing-relaxing techniques; responsibilities of spouse, family member, or friend who will be accompanying woman through labor and delivery; and care of newborn, including clothing, feeding and daily hygienic care

Complies with care

As stated earlier

Demonstrates relaxation, breathing techniques, and other techniques to be used in labor as taught in prenatal education classes or by prenatal nurse

Demonstrates preparation of nipples for breast feeding

Discusses plans for care of newborn, help at home, preparation of siblings

Continued

Fetal well-being	FHR heard by dopptone at wk 12, by fetoscope by wk 24	FHR and rhythm are normal (120 to 160 beats/min) and regular; will be less if fetus is asleep and greater with fetal movement
	Fetal movements felt at 17 to 19 wk (quickening)	Fetal movements increase with maternal movements, may lessen during fetal sleep; same pattern of movements every 24 hr
		Height of fundus, abdominal growth, and estimation of weight within normal limits for the estimated gestational age; presentation size of infant and maternal pelvic configuration permit vaginal delivery
		Engagement occurs about 2 wk before term in nullipara; may not occur until labor is well established in parous women

Immunization Schedules for Children

Recommended schedule for active immunization of normal infants and children

Recommended Age	Immunization(s)*	Comments
2 mo	DTP, OPV	Can be initiated as early as 2 weeks of age in areas of high endemicity or during epidemics
4 mo	DTP, OPV	Two-month interval desired for OPV to avoid interference from previous dose
6 mo	DTP (OPV)	OPV is optional (may be given in areas with increased risk of polio exposure)
15 mo	Measles, mumps, rubella, (MMR)	MMR preferred to individual vaccines; tuberculin testing may be done
18 mo	DTP,†‡ OPV‡	
24 mo	HBPV	
4 to 6 yr§	DTP, OPV	At or before school entry
14 to 16 yr	Td	Repeat every 10 years throughout life

*DTP, diphtheria and tetanus toxoids with pertussis vaccine; HBPV, Haemophilus influenzae type b polysaccharide vaccine; MMR, live measles, mumps, and rubella viruses in a combined vaccine; OPV, oral poliovirus vaccine containing attenuated poliovirus types 1, 2, and 3; Td, adult tetanus toxoid (full dose) and diphtheria toxoid (reduced dose) in combination.

†Should be given 6 to 12 months after the third dose.

‡May be given simultaneously with MMR at 15 months of age.

§Up to the seventh birthday.

From American Academy of Pediatrics: Report of the committee on infectious diseases, ed 20, Elk Grove Village, Ill, 1986, The Academy.

Recommended immunization schedules for children not immunized in first year of life

Recommended Time	Immunization (s)*	Comments
Younger Than 7 years of Age		
First visit	DTP, OPV, MMR	MMR if child ≥15 months old; tuberculin testing may be done
Interval after first visit		
1 mo	HBPV†	For children 24-60 months
2 mo	DTP, OPV	
4 mo	DTP (OPV)	OPV is optional (may be given in areas with increased risk of poliovirus exposure)
10 to 16 mo	DTP, OPV	OPV is not given if third dose was given earlier

*DTP, diphtheria and tetanus toxoids with pertussis vaccine; HBPV, Haemophilus influenzae type b polysaccharide vaccine; MMR, live measles, mumps, and rubella viruses in combined vaccine; OPV, oral poliovirus vaccine; Td, tetanus toxoid and diphtheria toxoid.

†Haemophilus influenzae type b polysaccharide vaccine can be given, if necessary, simultaneously with DTP (at separate sites). The initial three doses of DTP can be given at 1- to 2-month intervals; so, for the child in whom immunization is initiated at 24 months old or older, one visit could be eliminated by giving DTP, OPV, MMR at the first visit; DTP and HBPV at the second visit (1 month later); and DTP and OPV at the third visit (2 months after the first visit). Subsequent DTP and OPV 10 to 16 months after the first visit are still indicated.

From American Academy of Pediatrics: Report of committee on infectious diseases, ed 20, Elk Grove Village, Ill, 1986, The Academy.

Continued.

Recommended immunization schedules for children not immunized in first year of life—cont'd

Recommended Time	Immunization(s)*	Comments
4 to 6 yr (at or before school entry)	DTP, OPV	DTP is not necessary if the fourth dose was given after the fourth birthday; OPV is not necessary if recommended OPV dose at 10-16 months following first visit was given after the fourth birthday
Age 14 to 16 yr	Td	Repeat every 10 years throughout life
7 Years of Age and Older		
First visit	Td, OPV, MMR	
Interval after first visit		
2 mo	Td, OPV	
8 to 14 mo	Td, OPV	
Age 14 to 16 yr	Td	Repeat every 10 years throughout life

Burn
Charts

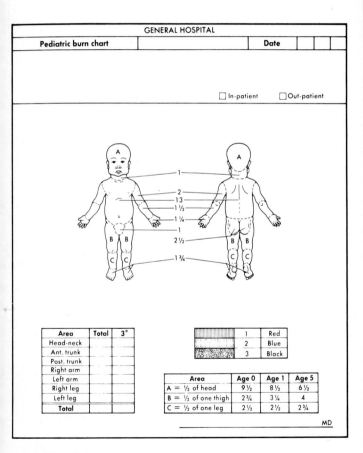

Pediatric burn chart.
(From Sheehy SB and Barber J: Emergency nursing principles and practice, ed 2, St Louis, 1985, The CV Mosby Co.)

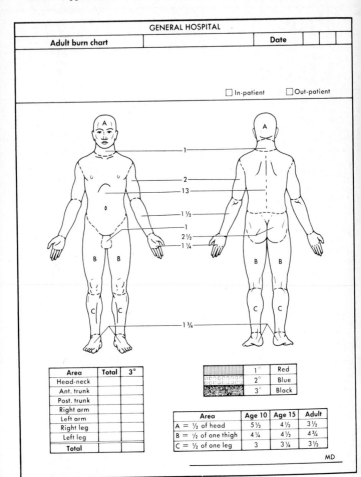

Adult burn chart

(From Sheehy SB and Barber J: Emergency nursing principles and practice, ed 2, St. Louis, 1985, The CV Mosby Co.)

Normal
References
Laboratory Values

Blood, plasma, or serum values

Determination	Reference Range	
	Conventional	SI*
Acetoacetate plus acetone	0.3-2.0 mg/100 ml	3-20 mg/l
Aldolase	1.3-8.2 mU/ml	12-75 nmol · s⁻¹/l
Alpha amino nitrogen	3.0-5.5 mg/100 ml	2.1-3.9 mmol/l
Ammonia	80-110 µg/100 ml	47-65 µmol/l
Ascorbic acid	0.4-1.5 mg/100 ml	23-85 µmol/l
Barbiturate	0	0 µmol/l
	Coma level: phenobarbital, approximately 10 mg/100 ml; most other drugs, 1-3 mg per 100 ml	
Bilirubin (van den Bergh test)	One minute: 0.4 mg/100 ml	Up to 7 µmol/l
	Direct: 0.4 mg/100 ml	Up to 17 µmol/l
	Total: 1.0 mg/100 ml	
	Indirect is total minus direct	
Blood volume	8.5-9.0% ob doby weight in kg	80-85 ml/kg
Bromide	0	0 mmol/l
	Toxic level: 17 mEq/l	

Bromsulfalein (BSP)	Less than 5% retention 45 min after 5 mg/kg IV	<0.05 1
Calcium	8.5-10.5 mg/100 ml (slightly higher in children)	2.1-2.6 mmol/l
Carbon dioxide content	24-30 mEq/l; 20-26 mEq/l in infants (as HCO_3^-)	24-30 mmol/l
Carbon monoxide	Symptoms with over 20% saturation	0 (1)
Carotenoids	0.8-4.0 µg/ml	1.5-7.4 µmol/l
Ceruloplasmin	27-37 mg/100 ml	1.8-2.5 µmol/l
Chloride	100-106 mEq/l	100-106 mmol/l
Cholinesterase (pseudocholinesterase)	0.5 pH U or more/h; 0.7 pH U or more/h for packed cells	0.5 or more arb, unit
Copper	Total: 100-200 µg/100 ml	16-31 µmol/l
Creatine phosphokinase (CPK)	Female 5-35 mU/ml; Male 5-55 mU/ml	$0.08-0.58$ µmol · s^{-1} l
Creatinine	0.6-1.5 mg/100 ml	60-130 µmol/l
Ethanol	0.3%-0.4%, marked intoxication; 0.4%-0.5%, alcoholic stupor; 0.5% or over, alcoholic coma	65-87 mmol/l; 87-109 mmol/l; >109 mmol/l
Glucose	Fasting: 70-100 mg/100 ml	3.9-5.6 mmol/l

Continued.

Adapted by permission from the New England Journal of Medicine, Vol. 302, pages 37-48, 1980.
*Abbreviations used: SI, Système international d'Unités (The SI for the health professions. World Health Organization, Office of Publications, Geneva, 1977); d, 24 hours; P, plasma; S, serum; B, blood; U, urine; l, liter; h, hour; and s, second.

Blood, plasma, or serum values—cont'd

Determination	Reference Range	
	Conventional	SI
Iron	50-150 μg/100 ml (higher in males)	9.0-26.9 μmol/l
Iron binding capacity	250-410 μg/100 ml	44.8-73.4 μmol/l
Lactic acid	0.6-1.8 mEq/l	0.6-1.8 mmol/l
Lactic dehydrogenase	60-120 U/ml	1.00-2.00 μmol · s^{-1}/l
Lead	50 μg/100 ml or less	Up to 2.4 μmol/l
Lipase	2 U/ml or less	Up to 2 arb. unit
Lipids		
Cholesterol	120-220 mg/100 ml	3.10-5.69 mmol/l
Cholesterol esters	60%-70% of cholesterol	
Phospholipids	9-16 mg/100 ml as lipid phosphorus	2.9-5.2 mmol/l
Total fatty acids	190-420 mg/100 ml	1.9-4.2 g/l
Total lipids	450-1000 mg/100 ml	4.5-10.0 g/l
Triglycerides	40-150 mg/100 ml	0.4-1.5 g/l
Lithium	Toxic level 2 mEq/l	2 mmol/l
Magnesium	1.5-2.0 mEq/l	0.8-1.3 mmol/l
5′Nucleotidase	0.3-3.2 Bodansky U	30-290 nmol · s^{-1}/l
Osmolality	285-295 mOsm/kg water	285-295 mmol/kg
Oxygen saturation (arterial)	96%-100%	0.96-1.00 1
P_{CO_2}	35-43 mm Hg	4.7-6.0 kPa

pH	7.35-7.45	Same
Po₂	75-100 mm Hg (dependent on age) while breathing room air	10.0-13.3 kPa
	Above 500 mm Hg while on 100% O₂	
Phenylalanine	0.2 mg/100 ml	0.120 μmol/l
Phenytoin (dilantin)	Therapeutic level, 5-20 μg/ml	19.8-79.5 μmol/l
Phosphorus (inorganic)	3.0-4.5 mg/100 ml (infants in 1st year up to 6.0 mg/100 ml)	1.0-1.5 mmol/l
Potassium	3.5-5.0 mEq/l	3.5-5.0 mmol/l
Primidone (Mysoline)	Therapeutic level 4-12 μg/ml	18-55 μmol/l
Protein: Total	6.0-8.4 g/100 ml	60-84 g/l
Albumin	3.5-5.0 g/100 ml	35-50 g/l
Globulin	2.3-3.5 g/100 ml	23-35 g/l
Electrophoresis	*% of total protein*	*Of total protein*
Albumin	52-68	0.52-0.68
Globulin:		
Alpha₁	4.2-7.2	0.042-0.072
Alpha₂	6.8-12	0.068-0.12
Beta	9.3-15	0.093-0.15
Gamma	13-23	0.13-0.23
Pyruvic acid	0-0.11 mEq/l	0-0.11 mmol/l
Quinidine	Therapeutic: 1.5-3 μg/ml	4.6-9.2 μmol/l
	Toxic: 5-6 μg/ml	15.4-18.5 μmol/l

Continued.

Blood, plasma, or serum values—cont'd

Determination	Reference Range	
	Conventional	SI
Salicylate:	0	
Therapeutic	20-25 mg/100 ml;	1.4-1.8 mmol/l
	25-30 mg/100 ml to age 10 yrs. 3 h post dose	1.8-2.2 mmol/l
Toxic	More than 30 mg/100 ml over 20 mg 100 ml after age 60	Over 2.2 mmol/l Over 1.4 mmol/l
Sodium	135-145 mEq/l	135-145 mmol/l
Sulfate	0.5-1.5 mg/100 ml	0.05-1.2 mmol/l
Sulfonamide	0 mg/100 ml	0 mmol/l
Transaminase (SGOT) (aspartate aminotransferase)	Therapeutic: 5-15 mg/100 ml 10-40 U/ml	0.08-0.32 µmol · s^{-1}/l
Urea nitrogen (BUN)	8-25 mg/100 ml	2.9-8.9 mmol/l
Uric acid	3.0-7.0 mg/100 ml	0.18-0.42 mmol/l
Vitamin A	0.15-0.6 µg/ml	0.5-2.1 µmol/l
Vitamin A tolerance test	Rise to twice fasting level in 3 to 5 h	

Urine values

Determination	Reference Range	
	Conventional	SI
Acetone plus acetoacetate (quantitative)	0	0 mg/l
Alpha amino nitrogen	64-199 mg/d; not more than 1.5% of total nitrogen	4.6-14.2 mmol/d
Amylase	24-76 U.ml	24-76 arb. unit
Calcium	150 mg/d or less	3.8 or less mmol/d
Catecholamines	Epinephrine: 20 μg/d less than	<55 nmol/d
	Norepinephrine: less than 100 μg/d	<590 nmol/d
Copper	0-100 μg;d	0-1.6 μmol/d
Coproporphyrin	50-250 μg/d	80-380 nmol/d
	Children less than 80 lb 0-75 μg/d	0-115 nmol/d
Creatine	Less than 100 mg/d or less than 6% of creatinine. In pregnancy up to 12%. In children younger than 1 yr.: may equal creatinine. In older children: up to 30% of creatinine	<0.75 mmol/d
Cystine or cysteine	0	0

Continued.

Urine values—cont'd

Determination	Reference Range	
	Conventional	SI
Follicle-stimulating hormone:		
Follicular phase	5-20 IU/d	Same
Mid-cycle	15-60 IU/d	
Luteal phase	5-15 IU/d	
Monopausal	50-100 IU/d	
Men	5-25 IU/d	
Hemoglobin and myoglobin	0	
5-Hydroxyindole acetic acid	2-9 mg/d (women lower than men)	10-45 µmol/d
Lead	0.08 µg/ml or 120 µg or less/d	0.39 µmol/l or less
Phenosulfonphthalein (PSP)	At least 25% excreted by 15 min; 40% by 30 min; 60% by 120 min	0.251
Phosphorus (inorganic)	Varies with intake; average 1 g/d	32 mmol/d
Porphobilinogen	0	0
Protein:		
Quantitative	<150 mg/24 h	<0.15 g/d

Steroids:
17-Ketosteroids (per day)

Age (yr)	Male (mg)	Female (mg)	Male (μmol/d)	Female (μmol/d)
10	1-4	1-4	3-14	3-14
20	6-21	4-16	21-73	14-56
30	8-26	4-14	28-90	14-49
50	5-18	3-9	17-62	10-31
70	2-10	1-7	7-35	3-24

17-Hydroxysteroids   3-8 mg/d (women lower than men)   8-22 μmol/d as hydrocortisone

Sugar:

Quantitative glucose	0	0 mmol/l
Identification of reducing substances		
Fructose	0	0 mmol/l
Pentose	0	0 mmol/l
Titratable acidity	20-40 mEq/d	20-40 mmol/d
Urobilinogen	Up to 1.0 Ehrlich U	To 1.0 arb. unit
Uroporphyrin	0	0 nmol/d
Vanillylmandelic acid (VMA)	Up to 9 mg/24 h	Up to 45 μmol/d

Special endocrine tests

Determination	Reference Range	
	Conventional	SI
Steroid Hormones		
Aldosterone		
Fasting, at rest, 210 mEq sodium diet	Excretion: 5-19 μg/24 h	14-53 nmol/d
	Supine: 48 ± 29 pg/ml	133 ± 80 pmol/l
	Upright: (2 h) 65 ± 23 pg/ml	180 ± 64 pmol/l
Fasting, at rest, 110 mEq sodium diet	Supine: 107 ± 45 pg/ml	279 ± 125 pmol/l
	Upright: (2 h) 239 ± 123 pg/ml	663 ± 341 pmol/l
Fasting, at rest, 10 mEq sodium diet	Supine: 175 ± 75 pg/ml	485 ± 208 pmol/l
	Upright: (2 h) 532 ± 228 pg/ml	1476 ± 632 pmol/l
Cortisol		
Fasting	8 a.m.: 5-25 μg/; 100 ml	0.14-0.69 μmol/l
At rest	8 p.m.: Below 10 μg/100 ml	0-0.28 μmol/l
20 U ACTH	4 h ACTH test: 30-45 μg/100 ml	0.83-1.24 μmol/l
Dexamethasone at midnight	Overnight suppression test: Less than 5 μg/100 ml	<0.14 nmol/l
11-Deoxycortisol	Excretion: 20-70 μg/24 h	55-193 nmol/d
	Responsive: More than 7.5 μg/100 ml (after metyrapone)	>0.22 μmol/l

Testosterone	Adult male: 300-1100 ng/100 ml	10.4-38.1 1 nmol/l
	Adolescent male: More than 100 ng/100 ml	>3.5 nmol/l
Unbound testosterone	Adult male: 3.06-24.0 ng/100 ml	106-832 pmol/l
	Adult female: 0.09-1.28 ng/100 ml	3.1-44.4 pmol/l
Polypeptide Hormones		
Adrenocorticotropin (ACTH)	15-70 pg/ml	3.3-15.4 pmol/l
Calcitonin	Undetectable in normals. >100 pg/ml in medullary carcinoma	0
		>29.3 pmol/l
Growth hormone		
Fasting, at rest	Less than 5 ng/ml	<233 pmol/l
After exercise	Children: More than 10 ng/ml	>465 pmol/l
	Male: Less than 5 ng/ml	<233 pmol/l
	Female: Up to 30 ng/ml	0-1395 pmol/l
After glucose	Male: Less than 5 ng/ml	<233 pmol/l
	Female: Less than 10 ng/ml	0-465 pmol/l
Insulin		
Fasting	6-26 μU/ml	43-187 pmol/l
During hypoglycemia	Less than 20 μU/ml	<144 pmol/l
After glucose	Up to 150 μU/ml	0-1078 pmol/l

Continued.

Special endocrine tests—cont'd

Determination	Reference Range		
	Conventional		SI
Luteinizing hormone			
Pre- or postovulatory	Male: 6-18 mU/ml		6-18 u/l
Midcycle peak	Female: 5-22 mU/ml		5-22 u/l
Parathyroid hormone	30-250 mU/ml		30-250 u/l
Prolactin	<10 μl equiv/ml		<10 ml equiv/l
	2-15 ng/ml		0.08-6.0 nmol/l
Renin activity			
Normal diet	Supine: 1.1 ± 0.8 ng/ml/h		0.9 ± 0.6 (nmol/l)h
	Upright: 1.9 ± 1.7 ng/ml/h		1.5 ± 1.3 (nmol/l)h
Low-sodium diet	Supine: 2.7 ± 1.8 ng/ml/h		2.1 ± 1.4 (nmol/l)h
	Upright: 6.6 ± 2.5 ng/ml/h		5.1 ± 1.9 (nmol/l)h
Low-sodium diet	Diuretics: 10.0 ± 3.7 ng/ml/h		7.7 ± 2.9 (nmol/l)h
Thyroid Hormones			
Thyroid-stimulating-hormone (TSH)	0.5-3.5 μU/ml		0.5-3.5 mU/l
Thyroxine-binding globulin capacity	15-25 μT$_4$/100 ml		193-322 nmol/l
Total tri-iodothyronine by radioim-munoassay (T$_3$)	70-190 ng/100 ml		1.08-2.92 nmol/l
Total thyroxine by RIA (T$_4$)	4-12 μg/100 ml		52-154 nmol/l
T$_3$ resin uptake	25-35%		0.25-0.35
Free thyroxine index (FT$_4$I)	1-4 ng/100 ml		12.8-51-2 pmol/l

Hematologic values

Determination	Reference Range	
	Conventional	SI
Coagulation factors:		
Factor I (fibrinogen)	0.15-0.35 g/100 ml	4.0-10.0 μmol/l
Factor II (prothrombin)	60%-140%	0.60-1.40
Factor V (accelerator globulin)	60%-140%	0.60-1.40
Factor VII-X (proconvertin-Stuart)	70%-130%	0.70-1.30
Factor X (Stuart factor)	70%-130%	0.70-1.30
Factor VIII (antihemophilic globulin)	50%-200%	0.50-2.0
Factor IX (plasma thromboplatic cofactor)	60%-140%	0.60-1.40
Factor XI (plasma thromboplastic antecedent)	60%-140%	0.60-1.40
Factor XII (Hageman factor)	60%-140%	0.60-1.40
Coagulation screening tests:		
Bleeding time (Simplate)	3-9 min	180-540 s
Prothrombin time	Less than 2-s deviation from control	Less than 2-s deviation from control
Partial thromboplastin time (activated)	25-37 s	25-37 s
Whole-blood clot lysis	No clot lysis in 24 h	0/d

Continued.

Hematologic values—cont'd

Determination	Reference Range	
	Conventional	SI
Fibrinolytic studies:		
Euglobin lysis	No lysis in 2 h	0 (in 2 h)
Fibrinogen split products:	Negative reaction at greater than 1:4 dilution	0 (at >1:4 dilution)
Thrombin time	Control ± 5 s	Control ± 5 s
"Complete" blood count:		
Hematocrit	Male: 45%-52%	Male: 0.42-0.52
	Female: 37%-48%	Female: 0.37-0.48
Hemoglobin	Male: 13-18 g/100 ml	Male: 8.1-11.2 mmol/l
	Female: 12-16 g/100 ml	Female: 7.4-9.9 mmol/l
Leukocyte count	4300-10,800/mm^3	4.3-10.8 × 10^9/l
Erythrocyte count	4.2-5.9 million/mm^3	4.2-5.9 × 10^{12}/l
Mean corpuscular volume (MCV)	80-94 μm^3	80-94 fl
Mean corpuscular hemoglobin (MCH)	27-32 pg	1.7-2.0 fmol
Mean corpuscular hemoglobin concentration (MCHC)	32%-36%	19-22.8 mmol/l
Erythrocyte sedimentation rate (Westergren method)	Male: 1-13 mm/h	Male: 1-13 mm/h
	Female: 1-20 mm/h	Female: 1-20 mm/h

Erythrocyte enzymes:		
Glucose-6-hosphate dehydrogenase	5-15 u/gHb	5-15 U/g
Pyruvate kinase	13-17 U/gHb	13-17 U/g
Ferritin (serum)		
Iron deficiency	0-20 ng/ml	0-20 μg/l
Iron excess	Greater than 400 ng/l	>400 μg/l
Folic acid		
Normal	Greater than 1.9 ng/ml	>4.3 mmol/l
Boderline	1.0-1.9 ng/ml	2.3-4.3 mmol/l
Haptoglobin	100-300 mg/100 ml	1.0-3.0 g/l
Hemoglobin studies:		
Electrophoresis for A_2 hemoglobin	1.5-3.5%	0.015-0.035
Hemoglobin F (fetal hemoglobin)	Less than 2%	<0.02
Hemoglobin, met- and sulf-	0	0
Serum hemoglobin	2-3 mg/100 ml	1.2-1.9 μmol/l
Thermolabile hemoglobin	0	0
L.E. (Lupus erythrmeatosus) prepara-tion:		
Heparin as anticoagulant	0	0
Defibrinated blood	0	0
Leukocyte alkaline phosphatase:		
Quantitative method	15-40 mg of phosphorus liberated/h/10^{10} cells	15-40 mg/h

Continued.

Hematologic values—cont'd

Determination	Reference Range	
	Conventional	SI
Qualitative method	Males: 33-188 U	33-188 U
	Females (off contraceptive pill): 30-160 U	30-160 U
Muramidase	Serum, 3-7 µg/ml	3-7 mg/l
	Urine, 0-2 µg/ml	0.2 mg/l
Osmotic fragility of erythrocytes	Increased if hemolysis occurs in more than 0.5% NaCl; decreased if hemolysis is incomplete in 0.3% NaCl	
Peroxide hemolysis	Less than 10%	<0.10
Platelet count	150,000-350,000/mm^3	150-350 × 10^9/l
Platelet function tests		
Clot retraction	50%-100%/2h	0.50-1.00/2h
Platelet aggregation	Full response to ADP, epinephrine and collagen	1.0
Platelet factor 3	33-57 s	33-57 s
Reticulocyte count	0.5%-1.5% red cells	0.005-.015
Vitamin B$_{12}$	90-280 pg/ml (borderline: 70-90)	66-207 pmol/l (borderline: 52-66)

Cerebrospinal Fluid Values

Determination	Reference Range	
	Conventional	SI
Bilirubin	0	0 µmol/l
Chloride	120-130 mEq/l (20 mEq/l higher than serum)	
Albumin	Mean: 29.5 mg/100 ml ±2 SD: 11-48 mg/100 ml	0.295 g/l ±2 SD: 0.11-0.48
IgG	Mean: 4.3 mg/100 ml ±2 SD: 0-8.6 mg/100 ml	0.043 g/l ±2 SD: 0-0.086
Glucose	50-75 mg/100 ml (30%-50% less than blood)	2.8-4.2 mmol/l
Pressure (initial)	70-180 mm of water	70-80 arb. u.
Protein:		
Lumbar	15-45 mg/100 ml	0.15-0.45 g/l
Cisternal	15-25 mg/100 m	0.15-0.25 g/l
Ventricular	5-15 mg/100 ml	0.05-0.15 g/l

Miscellaneous values

Determination	Reference Range	
	Conventional	SI
Autoantibodies in serum		
Thyroid colloid and microsomal antigens	Absent	
Stomach parietal cells	Absent	
Smooth muscle	Absent	
Kidney mitochondria	Absent	
Rabbit renal collecting ducts	Absent	
Cytoplasm of ova, theca cells, testicular interstitial cells	Absent	
Skeletal muscle	Absent	
Adrenal gland	Absent	
Carcinoembryonic antigen (CEA) in blood	0-2.5 ng/ml, 97% healthy nonsmokers	0-2.5 μg/l, 97% healthy nonsmokers
Cryoprecipitable proteins in blood	0	0 arb. unit
Digitoxin in serum	17 ± 6 ng/ml	22 ± 7.8 nmol/l
Digoxin in serum		
0.25 mg/d	1.2 ± 0.4 ng/ml	1.54 ± 0.5 nmol/l
0.5 mg/d	1.5 ± 0.4 ng/ml	1.92 ± 0.5 nmol/l

Duodenal drainage:		
pH	5.5-7.5	5.5-7.5
Amylase	More than 1200 U/total sample	>1.2 arb. u
Trypsin	Values from 35% to 160% "normal"	0.35-1.60
Viscosity	3 min or less	180 s or less
Gastric analysis	Basal:	
	Females 2.0 ± 1.8 mEq/h	0.6 ± 0.5
	Males 3.0 ± 2.0 mEq/h	0.8 ± 0.6 μmol/s
	Maximal: (after histalog or gastrin)	
	Females 16 ± 5 mEq/h	4.4 ± 1.4 μmol/s
	Males 23 ± 5 mEq/h	6.4 ± 1.4 μmol/s
Gastrin-I in blood	0-200 pg/ml	0-95 pmol/l
Immunologic tests		
Alpha-feto-globulin	Abnormal if present	
Alpha 1-antitrypsin	200-400 mg/100 ml	2.0-4.0 g/l
Antinuclear antibodies	Positive if detected with serum diluted 1:10	
Anti-DNA antibodies	Less than 15 units/ml	
Complement, total hemolytic	150-250 U/ml	
C3	Range	
	55-120 mg/100 ml	0.55-1.2 g/l
C4	Range	
	20-50 mg/100 ml	0.2-0.5 g/l

Continued.

Miscellaneous values—cont'd

Determination	Reference Range		
	Conventional	SI
Immunoglobulins in blood:		
IgG	1140 mg/100 ml	11.4 g/l
	Range 540-1663	5.5-16.6 g/l
IgA	214 mg/100 ml	2.14 g/l
	Range 66-344	0.66-3.44 g/l
IgM	168 mg/100 ml	1.68 g/l
	Range 39-290	0.39-2.9 g/l
Viscosity	1.4-1.8 expressed as relative viscosity of serum compared to water	
Iontophoresis	Children: 0-40 mEq sodium/liter.	0-40 mmol/l
	Adults: 0-60 mEq sodium/l	0-60 mmol/l
Propranolol (includes bioactive 4-OH metabolite) in serum 4h after last dose	100-300 ng/ml	386-1158 nmo/l

Stool fat	Less than 5 g in 24 h or less than 4% of measured fat intake in 3-d period	<5 g/d
Stool nitrogen	Less than 2 g/d or 10% of urinary nitrogen	<2 g/d
Synovial fluid:		
Glucose	Not less than 20 mg/100 ml lower than simultaneously drawn blood sugar	See blood glucose mmol/l
Mucin	Type 1 or 2 Grades as: Type 1-tight clump Type 2-soft clump Type 3-soft clump that breaks up Type 4-cloudy, no clump	1-2 arb. u
D-Xylose absorption	5-8 g/5 h in urine 40 mg per 100 ml in blood 2 h after ingestion of 25 g of D-xylose	33-53 mmol 2.7 mmol/l

Index

B